Copyright © 2021 -All rights reserved.

No part of this book may be reproduced or transmitted in any form or by any means, electronic or mechanical, including photocopying and recording, or by any information storage and retrieval system, without permission in writing from the publisher. This is a work of fiction. Names, places, characters and incidents are either the product of the author's imagination or are used fictitiously, and any resemblance to any actual persons, living or dead, organizations, events or locales is entirely coincidental. The unauthorized reproduction or distribution of this copyrighted work is ilegal.

Please note the information contained within this document is for educational and entertainment purposes only. All effort has been executed to present accurate, up to date, reliable, complete information. No warranties of any kind are declared or implied. Readers acknowledge that the author is not engaged in the rendering of legal, financial, medical, or professional advice. The content within this book has been derived from various sources. Please consult a licensed professional before attempting any techniques outlined in this book. By reading this document, the reader agrees that under no circumstances is the author responsible for any losses, direct or indirect, that are incurred as a result of the use of the information contained within this document, including, but not limited to, errors, omissions, or inaccuracies.

CONTENTS

INTRODUCTION 5
    Chapter 1. Bake Easy with the Bread Machine 6
    Benefits of Home-Baked Bread 6
    Types of Bread Makers 6
    Benefits of a Bread Maker 6
    How to Use a Bread Maker? 7
    Bread Baking Time 8
CHAPTER 2. INGREDIENTS AND BASICS OF BAKING KETO BREAD 9
    Keto and Gluten 9
    Keto Flours 9
CHAPTER 3. TIPS FOR USING YOUR BREAD MAKER MORE SUCCESSFULLY ... 10
CHAPTER 4. SAVORY BREAD RECIPES 11
    Cream Cheese Bread 11
    Lemon Poppy Seed Bread 12
    Cauliflower and Garlic Bread 13
    Almond Meal Bread 14
    Macadamia Nut Bread 15
    3-Seed Bread 16
    Cheesy Garlic Bread 17
    Cumin Bread 18
    Rosemary Bread 19
    Sesame and Flax Seed Bread 20
    Bacon and Cheddar Bread 21
    Olive Bread 22
    Jalapeño Cheese Bread 23
    Dill and Cheddar Bread 24
    Italian Mozzarella and Cream Cheese Bread 25
    Sourdough Dough 26
    Cheddar and Herb Bread 27
    Vegetable Loaf 28
    Cheese and Bacon Bread 29
    Pumpkin Bread 30
    Keto Almond Pumpkin Quick Bread 31
    Keto Basil Parmesan Slices 32
CHAPTER 5. SWEET BREAD RECIPES 33
    Banana Bread 33
    Sweet Avocado Bread 34
    Coconut Milk Bread 35
    Chocolate, Mixed Berry, and Nuts Cake 36
    Cinnamon Bread 37
    Lemon Raspberry Loaf 38
    Walnut Bread 39
    Almond Butter Bread 40
    Chocolate Zucchini Bread 41

- Pumpkin Bread 42
- Strawberry Bread 43
- Cranberry and Orange Bread 44
- Blueberry Bread 45
- Chocolate Bread 46
- Delicious Lemon Bread 47
- Strawberry Bread 48
- Delicious Pumpkin Bread 49
- Delicious Cranberry and Cream Cheese 50
- Chocolate Bread 51
- Keto Apple Bread 52
- Low-Carb Cranberry and Walnut Bread 53
- Chocolate and Pistachio Bread 54
- Low-Carb Date and Walnut Bread 55
- Buttermilk Bread 56
- Peach Cake Bread 57
- Garlic and Dill Bread 58
- Chocolate, Mixed Berry, and Nuts Bread 59
- Low-Carb Wheat-Style Bread 60
- Lemon and Blueberry Bread 61
- Orange Bread 62
- Low-Carb Pound Cake Loaf 63
- Red Velvet Cake 64
- Vegan Keto Bread 65
- Zucchini Bread 66
- Raspberry Bread 67
- Blueberry Bread 68
- Chocolate Bread 69
- Banana Bread 70
- Avocado Bread 71
- Gingerbread Cake 72
- Lemon Bread 73
- Holiday Bread 74
- American Cheese Beer Bread 75
- Date and Walnut Bread 76

CHAPTER 6. MORE BREAD RECIPES 77
- Basil Cheese Bread 77
- Cheese Sausage Bread 78
- French Ham Bread 79
- Keto Onion Bread 80
- Tomato Bread 81
- Keto Basil Parmesan Slices 82
- Zucchini Bread 83
- Bacon Bread 84
- Cauliflower Bread 85
- Herb Bread 86

Cream Cheese Bread 87
Garlic Bread 88
Sesame Bread 89
Scandinavian Bread 90
Feta Oregano Bread 91
Cottage Cheese Bread 92
Parmesan Cheddar Bread 93
Pepper Cheddar Bread 94
Olive Cheese Bread 95
Goat Cheese Bread 96
Pumpkin Pecan Bread 97
Ricotta Chive Bread 98
Cheese Cauliflower Broccoli Bread 99
Anise Almond Bread 100
Cinnamon Cake 101
Collagen Keto Bread 102
APPENDIX : RECIPES INDEX 103

INTRODUCTION

As a beginner, starting a Ketogenic diet lifestyle can be challenging, especially without proper guidance. The Keto diet is beneficial for your health and wellbeing. However, bread lovers often find it hard to maintain the diet because of the lack of delicious low-carb bread options. This cookbook will make it possible for you to follow the keto diet and not give up the foods you love. The recipes in this book will help you eat all your favorite bread while remaining in ketosis. In this keto bread machine book, you will find your favorite keto bread recipes.

The relationship between humans and bread as food is mystical. If you love bread but struggling to find easy keto bread machine bread recipes, then this bread machine cookbook is for you. When following a keto diet, it is highly recommended that you do not eat carb-rich foods like bread again. This book will allow you to eat healthily and, at the same time, permit you to maintain your very hectic schedule. If you want to lose belly fat without stopping eating bread, then this keto bread machine cookbook is perfect for you. This keto bread machine recipe book includes low-carb bread recipes for perfect keto baking.

Even if you haven't used a bread machine before, you do not have to worry because bread machines are simple to use and extremely user-friendly. Soon, bread machine will become a truly essential and irreplaceable help in your kitchen. All the recipes are really easy-to-follow, and you can cook them with your kids. With this keto bread maker cookbook, you just buy easy-to-find ingredients, put them in the bread machine, and enjoy delicious low-carb bread a little while later. The bread recipes are great for sandwiches, toasts, and as a separate snack. These recipes can make your culinary experience fun again!

Chapter 1. Bake Easy with the Bread Machine
Benefits of Home-Baked Bread

1. Lower cost: Baking your own bread can help you lower the cost.
2. Better taste: You bake your own bread. You can adjust bread ingredients and make the bread tastier.
3. More nutrition: Store bought bread is not nutrition-rich. Store bought bread offers more filler ingredients and less nutrition. On the other hand, home-baked bread is more nutritious.
4. Custom recipes: You can adjust recipes and create bread from custom recipes.
5. Enjoyment: You can enjoy the whole process of baking warm, flavorful, and delicious bread in your home.
6. Fresh: Homemade bread is guaranteed fresh. You are making your own bread, so it is always fresh.
7. No preservatives: Usually, store-bought bread has harmful ingredients. By baking at home, you can avoid these preservatives.

Types of Bread Makers

There are a variety of bread machines available in the market today:
1. Vertical bread maker. This type of bread machine is used for baking loaves in a vertical manner, which is how the bread pan is positioned and shaped. This type of bread machine has one kneading paddle.
2. Horizontal bread maker: This type of bread maker is used for baking loaves that are horizontally shaped and are most common in commercial bread making.
3. Small bread maker: Small bread makers are most ideal for use in your small home kitchen. This is ideal for a family setting.
4. Large bread maker: This type of bread maker is ideal when baking for a large group of people.
5. Gluten-free bread maker: This type of bread maker has a setting for gluten-free bread built in it.

Benefits of a Bread Maker

1. You get to enjoy freshly-baked bread right in the comfort of your home. The taste is also rich and full of flavor.
2. Most bread makers have a timer feature where you can set it to bake in the morning, and when you wake up, you can have warm bread for your breakfast.
3. You get to be in charge of what you eat since you get to select the ingredients you want to use in your bread. This is ideal for those how to have food allergies or want to eat certain types of foods and refrain from other types.

4. Baking bread using a bread maker is easy. All you have to do is mix your ingredients, put them into the bread pan, and select your setting option.
5. A bread maker can be a long-term money saver. This is especially true if you prefer certain types of special bread with specific ingredients.
6. Bread makers are built in such a way that you get to bake certain types of bread, depending on your needs.
7. The bread machines consume a low amount of electricity compared to the oven. So you save on the electricity bill.
8. Another important advantage is that you avoid the fatigue of having to do everything manually. All you have to do is prepare and weigh the ingredients. Then place them in the bread machine pan in the order indicated by the recipe and press one or more buttons. Then the bread machine will do all the rest from creating the dough to the fermentation and then the final cooking.
9. Easy to use: Bread makers available in the market are automatic. This feature of bread makers provides convenience to its users.
10. Allows for multi-tasking: Bread machines allow users to multi-task. You can do other household chores while the bread machine bakes the bread.

How to Use a Bread Maker?

The primary techniques used in making bread using a bread machine are:
• Mixing and resting: The ingredients are mixed together well and then allowed to rest before kneading.
• Kneading: Kneads, squishes, stretches, turns, and presses the dough for 20 to 30 minutes, depending on the machine and setting.
• First rise: This is also called bulk fermentation.
• Stir down: (1 and 2). The paddles rotate to bring the loaf down and redistribute the dough before the second and third rise.
• Second and third rise: The second rise is about 15 minutes. At the end of the third rise (15-30 minutes), the loaf will almost double in size.
• Baking: There will be one final growth spurt for the yeast in the dough in the first 4 minutes or so of the baking process before the bread bakes into the finished loaf.

<u>Cycles and Settings</u>
1. Basic: This is the most commonly used setting. It is often used for traditional white loaves.
2. Whole wheat: If you are making a bread that uses whole wheat flour, then this is the setting you will use. Whole wheat flour requires a longer bake time.
3. Gluten-free: Use this setting for gluten-free recipes.
4. Sweetbread: This setting is used for most sweet bread recipes that include yeast.
5. French bread: This setting is used for French breads and artisan breads.

6. Quick/Rapid: These breads will bake quickly and have short rise times.
7. Quick Bread: This setting is used for most breads that require no rising times and are baked immediately.
8. Jam: Some bread machines will offer special settings such as jam. This setting allows you to make your own homemade jam.
9. Dough: This is another specialty setting to create the dough.
10. Other/Custom: This setting allows you to use customized settings.

Bread Baking Time

Bread Type Time

Basic	3:25 hours
Sweet	3:27 hours
Whole Wheat	3:48 hours
French	3:35 hours
Gluten-free	2:10 hours
Quick/Rapid	1:20 hours
Express Bake	58 minutes
Jam	1:05 hour
Dough	1:30 hour
Pasta dough	14 minutes
Cake	1:30 hour
Bake	1 hour

The baking time can vary considerably among models.

How to Clean a Bread Maker?
• Clean your bread maker each time you use it.
• Never pour water or other types of fluid into the bread maker during cleaning. Just the bread tin is intended to have fluids inside.
• Unplug the machine then cool it before doing any cleaning.

Cleaning a Bread machine
1. Read the manual to know how to clean your bread machine. Unplug the bread machine and cool it completely. Remove all the residue and crumbs from the bread tin and then clean it.
2. Make sure everything is dry before using your bread machine again.

CHAPTER 2. INGREDIENTS AND BASICS OF BAKING KETO BREAD

Keto and Gluten

Gluten is a protein found in wheat and grains that enhances the elasticity of ground flours and causes them to rise (proof). It is the gluten that gives the bread its chewy texture and prevents it from crumbling after the baking process. Usually, when you remove the gluten factor from these flours, you also lose the properties that make bread and cakes what they are. Your baked products won't rise without gluten.
Is keto gluten-free?
Since gluten is mostly present in wheat and grains, the keto diet is totally gluten-free. All grain items are forbidden in the keto world.

Keto Flours

Almond flour
It is a low-carb flour, rich in minerals and vitamins. Tips on making almond flour:
• Use only dried or cool almonds.
• Grind a small quality of almonds at a time.
• Don't grind a portion for over thirty seconds.
• Slightly shake the blender or grinder as you go.

Coconut flour
• Coconut flour is rich in protein, fiber, and iron.
• Always sift the flour before using it.
• Mix dough more thoroughly then with usual flour.
• Watch the baking time.

Almond meal
Almond meal is also known as ground almonds.

Chocolate and coconut products
Use dark chocolate bars when baking.

Fruits
Use low-carb fruit options, such as berries.

Nuts
You can use macadamia, walnuts, and pecans.

Pumpkin seed/Sunflower seed meal
Use a food processor or coffee grinder to make your own homemade pumpkin seed or sunflower meals.

Flax meal
Flaxseed or ground flax is a very nourishing and a great source of the nutrients.

Psyllium husk

Powdered psyllium makes for a dense bread.

Low-carb sweeteners

They include Natvia, Erythritol, Stevia, Xylitol, and Swerve.

CHAPTER 3. TIPS FOR USING YOUR BREAD MAKER MORE SUCCESSFULLY

Bread machine tips:
- You must read your bread machine's manual and understand how it works.
- Do not exceed the capacity of your bread machine pan. Even 1 tsp. could make a difference.
- Check your bread machine's instructions to know the proper order.
- Use room temperature eggs.
- Do not use a delayed mix cycle when using milk.
- Cut margarine or butter into small pieces before adding them into the machine.

More tips:

1. Start simple: If you are a beginner bread maker, then start with simple recipes.
2. Be careful about substitutions: As a beginner, strictly follow the recipes. Once you have a year of baking experience, then you can start experimenting. Same goes for the yeast. Different types of yeast will produce different results so do not substitute without being sure.
3. You can open the lid: Check the dough after 5 minutes of adding the ingredients. You may notice various things, such as
- You forgot to attach the blade.
- The dough is too moist. You need to add 1 tbsp. flour at a time to fix it.
- The dough is too dry. You need to add 1 tbsp. water at a time to fix it.
4. Know in which order you need to add ingredients to the machine. With most bread machines, you start with liquids then finish with dry ingredients.
5. Know the capacity of your machine.
6. You can use the basic cycle for most breads.
7. Never place the yeast in direct contact with sugar or salt. Create a shallow pocket in the top of the flour with a spoon and place the yeast there. Take care that the yeast doesn't come into contact with the liquid.
8. Use a whisk to aerate the flour. Then scoop the flour lightly into a dry measuring cup.

CHAPTER 4. SAVORY BREAD RECIPES

Cream Cheese Bread

Prep time: 10 minutes
Cook time: 4 hours
Servings: 12 slices

Ingredients
- ¼ cup butter, unsalted
- 1 cup and 3 tbsp. cream cheese, softened
- 4 egg yolks
- 1 tsp. vanilla extract
- 1 tsp. baking powder
- ¼ tsp. sea salt
- 2 tbsp. monk fruit powder
- ½ cup peanut flour

Directions
1. Add butter and cream cheese until combined. Then beat in egg yolks, vanilla, baking powder, salt, and monk fruit powder and mix well.
2. Add the egg mixture into the bread bucket. Top with flour and shut the lid.
3. Select the Basic/white cycle or low-carb setting and press Start.
4. Remove the bread when done.
5. Cool, slice, and serve.

Nutritional Facts Per Serving
- Calories: 98
- Fat: 7.9g
- Carb: 2.2g
- Protein: 3.5g

Lemon Poppy Seed Bread

Prep time: 10 minutes
Cook time: 4 hours
Servings: 6

Ingredients
- 3 eggs
- 1 ½ tbsp. butter, unsalted and melted
- 1 ½ tbsp. lemon juice
- 1 lemon, zested
- 1 ½ cups almond flour
- ¼ cup erythritol sweetener
- ¼ tsp. baking powder
- 1 tbsp. poppy seeds

Directions
1. Beat eggs, butter, lemon juice, and lemon zest until combined.
2. In another bowl, add flour, sweetener, baking powder, and poppy seeds and mix well.
3. Add the egg mixture into the bread pan, top with flour mixture, and cover.
4. Select the Basic/White cycle or low-car setting and press Start.
5. Remove the bread when done.
6. Cool, slice, and serve.

Nutritional Facts Per Serving
- Calories: 201
- Fat: 17.5g
- Carb: 2.8g
- Protein: 8.2g

Cauliflower and Garlic Bread

Prep time: 10 minutes
Cook time: 4 hours
Servings: 9

Ingredients
- 5 eggs, separated
- ⅔ cup coconut flour
- 1 ½ cup riced cauliflower
- 1 tsp. minced garlic
- ½ tsp. sea salt
- ½ tbsp. chopped rosemary
- ½ tbsp. chopped parsley
- ¾ tbsp. baking powder
- 3 tbsp. butter, unsalted

Directions
1. Place the cauliflower rice in a bowl and cover it. Microwave for 3 to 4 minutes or until steamed. Then drain. Wrap in a cheesecloth and remove as much moisture as possible. Set aside.
2. Place egg whites in a bowl and whisk until stiff peaks form.
3. Then transfer ¼ of the whipped egg whites into a food processor. Add remaining ingredients except for cauliflower and pulse for 2 minutes until blended.
4. Add cauliflower rice, and pulse for 2 minutes until combined. Then pulse in remaining egg whites until just mixed.
5. Add batter into the bread bucket and cover.
6. Select the Basic/white cycle or low-carb. Press Start.
7. Remove the bread when done.
8. Cool, slice, and serve.

Nutritional Facts Per Serving
- Calories: 108
- Fat: 8g
- Carb: 3g
- Protein: 6g

Almond Meal Bread

<u>Prep time: 10 minutes</u>
<u>Cook time: 4 hours</u>
<u>Servings: 10 slices</u>

Ingredients
- 4 eggs
- ¼ cup melted coconut oil
- 1 tbsp. apple cider vinegar
- 2 ¼ cups almond meal
- 1 tsp. baking soda
- ¼ cup ground flaxseed meal
- 1 tsp. onion powder
- 1 tbsp. minced garlic
- 1 tsp. sea salt
- 1 tsp. chopped sage leaves
- 1 tsp. fresh thyme
- 1 tsp. chopped rosemary leaves

Directions
1. In a bowl, beat eggs, coconut oil, and vinegar until mixed.
2. In another bowl, place an almond meal and add the remaining ingredients. Mix well.
3. Add the egg mixture into the bread bucket, and top with flour mixture. Cover the lid.
4. Select the Basic/White cycle or low-carb. Press Start.
5. Remove the bread when done.
6. Cool, slice, and serve.

Nutritional Facts Per Serving
- Calories: 104
- Fat: 8.8g
- Carb: 2.1g
- Protein: 4g

Macadamia Nut Bread

Prep time: 10 minutes
Cook time: 4 hours
Servings: 8 slices

Ingredients
- 1 cup natural macadamia nut butter
- 5 eggs
- ½ tsp. apple cider vinegar
- ¼ cup coconut flour
- ½ tsp. baking soda

Directions
1. Mix macadamia nut butter, eggs, and vanilla and mix until smooth.
2. Stir in flour and baking soda and mix well.
3. Add the batter into the bread bucket and cover.
4. Select Basic/White cycle or low-carb. Press Start.
5. Remove the bread when done.
6. Cool, slice, and serve.

Nutritional Facts Per Serving
- Calories: 155
- Fat: 14.3g
- Carb: 3.9g
- Protein: 5.6g

3-Seed Bread

<u>Prep time: 10 minutes</u>
<u>Cook time: 4 hours</u>
<u>Servings: 18 slices</u>

Ingredients
- 2 eggs
- ¼ cup butter, melted
- 1 cup warm water (100F)
- ¼ cup chia seeds
- ½ cup pumpkin seeds
- ½ cup psyllium husks
- ½ cup sunflower seeds
- ¼ cup coconut flour
- ¼ tsp. salt
- 1 tsp. baking powder

Directions
1. Beat eggs and butter in a bowl until well blended.
2. Add flour to another bowl. Then stir in the remaining ingredients except for water until mixed.
3. Pour water into the bread bucket, add egg mixture, and top with flour mixture. Cover.
4. Select the Basic/White cycle or low-carb. Press Start.
5. Remove the bread when done.
6. Cool, slice, and serve.

Nutritional Facts Per Serving
- Calories: 139
- Fat: 10g
- Carb: 5.6g
- Protein: 5g

Cheesy Garlic Bread

Prep time: 10 minutes
Cook time: 4 hours
Servings: 16 slices

Ingredients
- 5 eggs
- 2 cups almond flour
- ½ tsp. xanthan gum
- 1 tsp. garlic powder
- 1 tsp. salt
- 1 tsp. parsley
- 1 tsp. Italian seasoning
- 1 tsp. dried oregano
- 1 stick of butter, unsalted and melted
- 1 cup grated mozzarella cheese
- 2 tbsp. ricotta cheese
- 1 cup, grated cheddar cheese
- ⅓ cup grated parmesan cheese

For topping
- ½ stick butter, unsalted and melted
- 1 tsp. garlic powder

Directions
1. Whisk the eggs in a bowl.
2. Place flour in another bowl. Stir in xanthan gum and all the cheeses until well combined.
3. Place butter in a bowl and add all the seasonings to it. Mix well.
4. Add the egg mixture into the bread bucket. Then add the seasoning mixture and flour mixture. Cover.
5. Select the Basic/white cycle or low-carb setting. Press Start.
6. Remove the bread when done.
7. Cool, slice, and serve.

Nutritional Facts Per Serving
- Calories: 250
- Fat: 14.5g
- Carb: 1.4g
- Protein: 7.2g

Cumin Bread

<u>Prep time: 10 minutes</u>
<u>Cook time: 4 hours</u>
<u>Servings: 12 slices</u>

Ingredients
- 2 eggs
- 1 ½ tbsp. avocado oil
- ⅔ cup coconut milk, unsweetened
- 2 tbsp. Picante sauce
- 1 cup almond flour
- ½ cup coconut flour
- ¼ tsp. salt
- 1 tbsp. baking powder
- ¼ tsp. mustard powder
- 2 tsp. ground cumin

Directions
1. Beat eggs until frothy, then beat in oil, milk, and sauce until combined.
2. In another bowl, place flours, then stir in remaining ingredients and mix.
3. Add egg mixture into the bread bucket, top with flour mixture, then cover.
4. Select the Basic/White cycle or low-carb. Press Start.
5. Remove the bread when done.
6. Cool, slices, and serve.

Nutritional Facts Per Serving
- Calories: 108
- Fat: 8.3g
- Carb: 4g
- Protein: 3.7g

Rosemary Bread

Prep time: 10 minutes
Cook time: 4 hours
Servings: 10 slices

Ingredients
- 6 eggs
- 8 tbsp. butter, unsalted and melted
- ½ cup, coconut flour
- 1 tsp. baking powder
- ¼ tsp. salt
- ½ tsp. onion powder
- 1 tsp. garlic powder
- 2 tsp. dried rosemary

Directions
1. Gently mix eggs and butter until well combined.
2. Place flour in another bowl. Stir in the remaining ingredients until mixed.
3. Add egg mixture into the bread bucket and top with flour mixture. Cover.
4. Select the Basic/White cycle or low-carb. Press Start.
5. Remove the bread when done.
6. Cool, slice, and serve.

Nutritional Facts Per Serving
- Calories: 147
- Fat: 12.5g
- Carb: 3.5g
- Protein: 4.6g

Sesame and Flax Seed Bread

Prep time: 10 minutes
Cook time: 4 minutes
Servings: 10 slices

Ingredients
- 3 eggs
- ½ cup cream cheese, softened
- 6 ½ tbsp. heavy whipping cream
- ¼ cup melted coconut oil
- ½ cup almond flour
- ¼ cup flaxseed
- 6 ½ tbsp. coconut flour
- 2 ⅔ tbsp. sesame seeds
- ½ tsp. salt
- 1 ½ tsp. baking powder
- 2 tbsp. ground psyllium husk powder
- ½ tsp. ground caraway seeds

Directions
1. Beat the eggs, cream cheese, whipping cream, and coconut oil until mixed.
2. Add flours in another bowl. Then stir in remaining ingredients and mix.
3. Add egg mixture into the bread bucket, then top with flour mixture. Cover.
4. Select the Basic/White cycle or low-carb. Press Start.
5. Remove the bread when done.
6. Cool, slice, and serve.

Nutritional Facts Per Serving
- Calories: 230
- Fat: 21g
- Carb: 6.2g
- Protein: 6.3g

Bacon and Cheddar Bread

Prep time: 10 minutes
Cook time: 4 hours
Servings: 9 slices

Ingredients
- 2 eggs
- ¼ cup beer
- 2 tbsp. butter, unsalted and melted
- ¼ cup bacon, cooked and crumbled
- ½ cup shredded cheddar cheese
- ½ tbsp. coconut flour
- 1 cup almond flour
- ¼ tsp. salt
- ½ tbsp. baking powder

Directions
1. Blend eggs, beer, and butter in a bowl. Fold in the bacon and cheese until just mixed.
2. Add egg mixture into the bread bucket. Top with flour mixture (flour mixed with dry ingredients) and cover.
3. Select the Basic/White cycle or low-carb and press Start.
4. Remove the bread when done.
5. Cool, slice, and serve.

Nutritional Facts Per Serving
- Calories: 140
- Fat: 12g
- Carb: 3g
- Protein: 5g

Olive Bread

Prep time: 10 minutes
Cook time: 4 hours
Servings: 10 slices

Ingredients
- 4 eggs
- 4 tbsp. avocado oil
- 1 tbsp. apple cider vinegar
- ½ cup coconut flour
- 1 tbsp. baking powder
- 2 tbsp. psyllium husk powder
- 1 ½ tbsp. dried rosemary
- ½ tsp. salt
- ⅓ cup black olives, chopped
- ½ cup boiling water

Directions
1. Beat eggs, then blend in oil. Stir in vinegar and fold in the olives.
2. In another bowl, place the flour, then stir in husk powder, baking powder, salt, and rosemary until mixed.
3. Add egg mixture into the bread bucket, top with flour mixture, and cover.
4. Select the Basic/White cycle or low-carb. Then press Start.
5. Remove the bread when done.
6. Cool, slice, and serve.

Nutritional Facts Per Serving
- Calories: 85
- Fat: 6.5g
- Carb: 3.4g
- Protein: 2g

Jalapeño Cheese Bread

Prep time: 10 minutes
Cook time: 4 hours
Servings: 8 slices

Ingredients
- 2 tbsp. Greek yogurt, full-fat
- 4 eggs
- ⅓ cup coconut flour
- ½ tsp. sea salt
- 2 tbsp. whole psyllium husks
- 1 tsp. baking powder
- ¼ cup diced, pickled jalapeños
- ¼ cup shredded cheddar cheese, divided

Directions
1. Beat yogurt and egg in a bowl.
2. Place the flour in another bowl. Add the remaining ingredients and mix well.
3. Add egg mixture into the bread bucket, top with flour mixture, and cover.
4. Select the Basic/White cycle or low-carb and press Start.
5. Remove the bread when done.
6. Cool, slice, and serve.

Nutritional Facts Per Serving
- Calories: 105
- Fat: 6.2g
- Carb: 3.4g
- Protein: 6.6g

Dill and Cheddar Bread

Prep time: 10 minutes
Cook time: 4 hours
Servings: 10 slices

Ingredients
- 4 eggs
- ¼ tsp. cream of tarter
- 5 tbsp. butter, unsalted
- 2 cups grated cheddar cheese
- 1 ½ cups almond flour
- 1 scoop of egg white protein
- ¼ tsp. salt
- 1 tsp. garlic powder
- 4 tsp. baking powder
- ¼ tbsp. dried dill weed

Directions
1. Beat eggs, cream of tartar, butter, and cheese until just mixed.
2. Place flour in another bowl. Then stir in egg white protein, salt, garlic powder, baking powder, and dill and mix.
3. Add the egg mixture into the bread bucket, top with flour mixture. Cover.
4. Select the Basic/White cycle or low-carb and press Start.
5. Remove the bread when done.
6. Cool, slice, and serve.

Nutritional Facts Per Serving
- Calories: 292
- Fat: 25.2g
- Carb: 6.1g
- Protein: 14.3g

Italian Mozzarella and Cream Cheese Bread

Prep time: 10 minutes
Cook time: 4 hours
Servings: 8 slices

Ingredients
- ¾ cup shredded mozzarella cheese
- ¼ cup cream cheese, softened
- 1 egg
- ⅓ cup almond flour
- ¼ tsp. garlic powder
- 2 tsp. baking powder
- ½ tsp. Italian seasoning
- ½ cup shredded cheddar cheese

Directions
1. Melt the mozzarella cheese and cream cheese in the microwave.
2. Beat the egg in another bowl.
3. Place flour in another bowl, add remaining ingredients, and mix.
4. Add blended egg into the bread bucket, top with melted cheese mixture, and then with flour mixture. Cover.
5. Select the Basic/White cycle or low-carb. Press Start.
6. Remove the bread when done.
7. Cool, slice, and serve.

Nutritional Facts Per Serving
- Calories: 171
- Fat: 14.5g
- Carb: 1.5g
- Protein: 3.3g

Sourdough Dough

<u>Prep time: 10 minutes</u>
<u>Cook time: 4 hours</u>
<u>Servings: 15</u>

Ingredients
- 2 eggs
- 6 egg whites
- ¾ cup coconut milk, unsweetened
- ¼ cup apple cider vinegar
- ½ cup of warm water (100F)
- 1 ½ cups almond flour
- ½ cup coconut flour
- ½ cup ground flaxseed
- 1 tsp. salt
- 1 tsp. baking soda
- ⅓ cup psyllium powder

Directions
1. In a bowl, add eggs, egg white, milk, vinegar, and water and whisk until combined.
2. In another bowl, place flour and stir in remaining ingredients until mixed.
3. Add the egg mixture into the bread bucket, top with flour mixture, and cover.
4. Select the Basic/White cycle or low-carb. Press Start.
5. Remove the bread when done.
6. Cool, slice, and serve.

Nutritional Facts Per Serving
- Calories: 115
- Fat: 8g
- Carb: 4.7g
- Protein: 5g

Cheddar and Herb Bread

Prep time: 10 minutes
Cook time: 4 hours
Servings: 16 slices

Ingredients
- 6 eggs
- ½ cup butter, unsalted, softened
- 2 cups almond flour
- 1 tsp. baking powder
- ½ tsp. xanthan gum
- 2 tbsp. garlic powder
- ½ tsp. salt
- 1 tbsp. dried parsley
- ½ tbsp. dried oregano
- 1 ½ cups shredded cheddar cheese

Directions
1. Beat eggs until frothy and then beat in the butter until combined.
2. Place flour in another bowl. Stir in remaining ingredients until mixed.
3. Add egg mixture into the bread bucket, top with flour mixture, and cover.
4. Select the Basic/White cycle or low-carb and press Start.
5. Remove the bread when done.
6. Cool, slice, and serve.

Nutritional Facts Per Serving
- Calories: 207
- Fat: 17.5g
- Carb: 5 g
- Protein: 7.2g

Vegetable Loaf

Prep time: 10 minutes
Cook time: 4 hours
Servings: 12 slices

Ingredients
- 4 eggs
- ¼ cup coconut oil
- 1 medium grated zucchini
- 1 cup grated pumpkin
- 1 small grated carrot
- ⅓ cup coconut flour
- 1 cup almond flour
- 2 tbsp. pumpkin seeds
- 2 tbsp. flax seeds
- 2 tbsp. sunflower seeds
- 2 tbsp. sesame seeds
- 2 tbsp. psyllium husks
- 2 tsp. salt
- 1 tbsp. smoked paprika
- 2 tsp. ground cumin
- 2 tsp. baking powder

Directions
1. Beat the eggs until frothy, beat in the oil, and then stir in zucchini, pumpkin, and carrot until just mixed.
2. Place flour in another bowl. Then stir in the remaining ingredients until mixed.
3. Add egg mixture into the bread bucket, top with flour mixture, and cover.
4. Select the Basic/White cycle or low-carb. Press Start.
5. Remove the bread when done.
6. Cool, slice, and serve.

Nutritional Facts Per Serving
- Calories: 181
- Fat: 15g
- Carb: 6.6g
- Protein: 6.9g

Cheese and Bacon Bread

Prep time: 10 minutes
Cook time: 3 hours and 25 minutes
Servings: 10 slices

Ingredients
- 7 ounces of diced bacon
- 1 ½ cups of almond flour
- 1 tbsp. of baking powder
- ⅓ cup of sour cream
- 2 large eggs
- 4 tbsp. of melted butter
- 1 cup of shredded cheddar cheese

Directions
1. Add in the flour, baking powder, sour cream, eggs, butter, and cheese in the bread machine.
2. Select White/Basic bread and press Start.
3. Check the dough after ten minutes.
4. Add the bacon after the beep.
5. Remove the bread when done.
6. Cool, slice, and serve.

Nutritional Facts Per Serving
- Calories: 176
- Fat: 26.25g
- Carb: 2.99g
- Protein: 14.44g

Pumpkin Bread

Prep time: 10 minutes
Cook time: 60 to 80 minutes
Servings: 12 slices

Ingredients
- 4 whole eggs
- 1 cup pumpkin puree
- 5 tbsp. unsalted butter/ghee, softened
- 2 tsp. apple cider vinegar
- 1 ⅓ cup almond flour
- ¼ cup coconut flour
- ¼ cup flaxseed meal
- 2 tbsp. psyllium husk powder
- 1 tbsp. pumpkin pie spice
- 1 tbsp. Keto baking powder
- ½ tsp. sea salt
- 1 cup allulose

For the glaze
- 1 tbsp. ginger, grated
- 1 tbsp. water
- 6 tbsp. xylitol
- 1 pinch sea salt

Directions
1. In a bowl, combine all the dry ingredients except the sweetener.
2. Carefully blend butter with the sweetener. Add eggs and vinegar.
3. Pour all the ingredients into the bread machine pan. Close the cover.
4. Select Cake (time depends on the bread machine – 60 to 80 minutes).
5. Press Start.
6. Remove the bread when done and cool.
7. Combine all the glaze ingredients in a bowl.
8. Cool the bread for 30 minutes, then spread the glaze on top.
9. Slice and serve.

Nutritional Facts Per Serving
- Calories: 177
- Fat: 13g
- Carb: 3g
- Protein: 5g

Keto Almond Pumpkin Quick Bread

Prep time: 10 minutes
Cook time: 60 minutes
Servings: 16

Ingredients
- ⅓ cup oil
- 3 large eggs
- 1 ½ cup pumpkin puree, canned
- 1 cup granulated sugar
- 1 ½ tsp. baking powder
- ½ tsp. baking soda
- ¼ tsp. salt
- ¾ tsp. ground cinnamon
- ¼ tsp. ground nutmeg
- ¼ tsp. ground ginger
- 3 cups almond flour
- ½ cup chopped pecans

Directions
1. Grease the bread machine pan with cooking spray. Mix all the wet ingredients in a bowl. Add all the dry ingredients except pecans until mixed.
2. Pour the batter onto your bread machine pan and place it back inside the bread machine. Close and select Quick Bread.
3. Add the pecans after the beep.
4. Remove the bread when done.
5. Cool, slice, and serve.

Nutritional Facts Per Serving
- Calories: 54
- Fat: 13.3g
- Carb: 6.3g
- Protein: 9.6g

Keto Basil Parmesan Slices

Prep time: 10 minutes
Cook time: 3 hours and 25 minutes
Servings: 16 slices

Ingredients
- 1 cup water
- ½ cup parmesan cheese, grated
- 3 tbsp. granulated sugar
- 1 tbsp. dried basil
- 1 ½ tbsp. olive oil
- 1 tsp. salt
- 3 cups almond flour
- 2 tsp. active dry yeast

Directions
1. Place everything in the bread machine according to bread machine recommendation.
2. Select Basic and press Start.
3. Remove the bread when done.
4. Cool, slice, and serve.

Nutritional Facts Per Serving
- Calories: 96
- Fat: 8g
- Carb: 7g
- Protein: 6g

CHAPTER 5. SWEET BREAD RECIPES

Banana Bread

Prep time: 10 minutes
Cook time: 4 hours
Servings: 12

Ingredients
- 2 eggs
- 1 tsp. banana extract
- ¼ cup erythritol sweetener
- 3 tbsp. butter, unsalted and softened
- 2 tbsp. almond milk, unsweetened
- 1 cup almond flour
- 2 tbsp. coconut flour
- ¼ cup walnuts, chopped
- 1 tsp. baking powder
- ¼ tsp. xanthan gum
- 1/8 tsp. sea salt
- 1 tsp. cinnamon

Directions
1. Beat the eggs with banana extract, sweetener, butter, and milk.
2. Place flours in another bowl, then stir in the remaining ingredients.
3. Add egg mixture into the bread bucket, top with flour mixture, and cover.
4. Select Basic/White cycle and press Start.
5. Remove the bread when done.
6. Cool, slice, and serve.

Nutritional Facts Per Serving
- Calories: 240
- Fat: 21g
- Carb: 6.8g
- Protein: 8.5g

Sweet Avocado Bread

Prep time: 10 minutes
Cook time: 4 hours
Servings: 12 slices

Ingredients
- 3 eggs
- 2 tbsp. erythritol sweetener
- 1 tbsp. vanilla extract
- 1 ½ cups mashed avocado
- 6 tbsp. coconut flour
- ¾ tsp baking soda
- ½ tsp. salt
- 2 tbsp. cocoa powder, unsweetened

Directions
1. Crack eggs in a bowl. Beat in sweetener and vanilla until fluffy and then mix in avocado.
2. Place flour in another bowl. Stir in the remaining ingredients until mixed.
3. Add egg mixture into the bread bucket and top with flour mixture. Cover.
4. Select Basic/White cycle or low-carb. Press Start.
5. Remove the bread when done.
6. Cool, slice, and serve.

Nutritional Facts Per Serving
- Calories: 94
- Fat: 6.1g
- Carb: 3.2g
- Protein: 4.2g

Coconut Milk Bread

Prep time: 10 minutes
Cook time: 3 hours and 25 minutes
Servings: 10

Ingredients
- 1 whole egg
- ½ cup lukewarm milk
- ½ cup lukewarm coconut milk
- ¼ cup butter, melted and cooled
- 1 tbsp. erythritol
- 4 cups almond flour, sifted
- 1 tbsp. active dry yeast
- 1 tsp. salt
- ½ cup coconut chips

Directions
1. Place everything in the bread machine, except for the coconut chips, according to bread machine recommendation.
2. Select Sweet and press Start.
3. Add the coconut chips into the dough after the beep.
4. Remove the bread when done.
5. Cool, slice, and serve.

Nutritional Facts Per Serving
- Calories: 124
- Fat: 15.3g
- Carb: 6g
- Protein: 9.5g

Chocolate, Mixed Berry, and Nuts Cake

Prep time: 10 minutes
Cook time: 3 hours and 25 minutes
Servings: 10 slices

Ingredients
- ½ cup of coconut flour
- 5 eggs
- ½ cup of erythritol
- ½ cup of unsalted butter
- ¼ tsp. of salt
- ½ tsp. of vanilla extract
- 3 tbsp. of coconut milk
- 1 cup of mixed berries of choice
- ⅓ cup of chopped pecans, walnuts, or almonds as desired
- ¼ cup of cocoa powder

Directions
1. Add everything in the bread machine except for the fruits and nuts.
2. Select Fruit bread and press Start.
3. Add the fruits and nuts after the beep.
4. Remove the bread when done.
5. Cool, slice, and serve.

Nutritional Facts Per Serving
- Calories: 165
- Fat: 14g
- Carb: 7g
- Protein: 4g

Cinnamon Bread

Prep time: 10 minutes
Cook time: 4 hours
Servings: 10

Ingredients
- 3 tbsp. sour cream
- 3 eggs
- 2 tsp. vanilla extract
- ¼ cup melted butter, unsalted
- 2 cups almond flour
- ⅓ cup erythritol sweetener
- 2 tbsp. cinnamon
- 1 tsp. baking soda
- 1 tsp. baking powder

Directions
1. Beat sour cream, eggs, vanilla, and butter until combined.
2. Place flour in another bowl and stir in sweetener, cinnamon, baking powder, and soda until mixed.
3. Add egg mixture into bread bucket, top with flour mixture, and cover.
4. Select Basic/White cycle and press Start.
5. Remove the bread when done.
6. Cool, slice, and serve.

Nutritional Facts Per Serving
- Calories: 169
- Fat: 14.5g
- Carb: 4.2g
- Protein: 5.4g

Lemon Raspberry Loaf

Prep time: 10 minutes
Cook time: 4 hours
Servings: 12

Ingredients
- 2 eggs
- 4 tbsp. sour cream
- 1 tsp. vanilla extract
- 1 tsp. lemon extract
- 4 tbsp. butter, unsalted and melted
- ¼ cup erythritol sweetener
- 2 tbsp. lemon juice
- ½ cup raspberries preserve
- 2 cup almond flour
- 1 ½ tsp. baking powder

Directions
1. Mix flour and baking powder in a bowl.
2. In another bowl, beat eggs, sour cream, extracts, butter, sweetener, and lemon juice until blended. Then stir in raspberry preserve and mix until just combined.
3. Add the egg mixture into the bread bucket, top with flour mixture, and cover.
4. Select Basic/White cycle and press Start.
5. Remove the bread when done.
6. Cool, slice, and serve.

Nutritional Facts Per Serving
- Calories: 171
- Fat: 14.3g
- Carb: 5g
- Protein: 4.6g

Walnut Bread

Prep time: 10 minutes
Cook time: 4 minutes
Servings: 10 slices

Ingredients
- 4 eggs
- 2 tbsp. apple cider vinegar
- 4 tbsp. coconut oil
- ½ cup lukewarm water
- 1 cup walnuts chopped
- ½ cup coconut flour
- 1 tbsp. baking powder
- 2 tbsp. psyllium husk powder
- ½ tsp. salt

Directions
1. Beat the eggs, vinegar, oil, and water until blended. Stir in the walnuts until just mixed.
2. In another bowl, place flour. Stir in baking powder, husk powder, and salt until mixed.
3. Add the egg mixture into the bread bucket, top with flour mixture, and cover.
4. Select Basic/White cycle and press Start.
5. Remove the bread when done.
6. Cool, slice, and serve.

Nutritional Facts Per Serving
- Calories: 201
- Fat: 8.1g
- Carb: 2.8g
- Protein: 6g

Almond Butter Bread

Prep time: 10 minutes
Cook time: 4 hours
Servings: 12 slices

Ingredients
- 3 eggs
- 1 cup almond butter
- 1 tbsp. apple cider vinegar
- ½ tsp. baking soda

Directions
1. Beat eggs, butter, vinegar, and baking soda in a bowl.
2. Add egg mixture into the bread bucket and cover.
3. Select the Basic/White cycle and press Start.
4. Remove the bread when done.
5. Cool, slice, and serve.

Nutritional Facts Per Serving
- Calories: 152
- Fat: 13g
- Carb: 5.6g
- Protein: 6.4g

Chocolate Zucchini Bread

Prep time: 10 minutes
Cook time: 4 hours
Servings: 14 slices

Ingredients
- 1 cup grated zucchini, moisture squeezed out thoroughly
- ⅓ cup ground flaxseed
- ½ cup almond flour
- ½ tsp. salt
- 2 ½ tsp. baking powder
- 1 ¼ tbsp. psyllium husk powder
- ⅓ cup cocoa powder
- 4 eggs
- 1 tbsp. coconut cream
- 5 tbsp. coconut oil
- ¾ cup erythritol sweetener
- 1 tsp. vanilla extract
- ½ cup sour cream
- ½ cup chocolate chips, unsweetened

Directions
1. In a bowl, place flaxseed and flour. Then stir in salt, grated zucchini, baking powder, husk, and cocoa powder until mixed.
2. In another bowl, beat the eggs, coconut cream, coconut oil, sweetener, and vanilla until combined.
3. Blend in half of the flour mixture, then add sour cream and remaining half of flour mixture until mixed, and fold in chocolate chips.
4. Add batter into the bread bucket and cover.
5. Select Basic/White cycle and press Start.
6. Remove the bread when done.
7. Cool, slice, and serve.

Nutritional Facts Per Serving
- Calories: 187
- Fat: 15.9g
- Carb: 3.6g
- Protein: 6.2g

Pumpkin Bread

Prep time: 10 minutes
Cook time: 4 hours
Servings: 12

Ingredients

- 2 eggs
- 1 cup almond butter, unsweetened
- ⅔ cup erythritol sweetener
- ⅔ cup pumpkin puree
- 1/8 tsp. ground cloves
- ½ tsp. ground cinnamon
- 1/8 tsp. ground ginger
- 1 tsp. baking powder
- ½ tsp. ground nutmeg

Directions

1. Crack eggs in a bowl. Then beat in remaining ingredients in the order described in the ingredients until mixed.
2. Add batter into the bread bucket and cover.
3. Select Basic/White cycle and press Start.
4. Remove the bread when done.
5. Cool, slice, and serve.

Nutritional Facts Per Serving

- Calories: 150
- Fat: 12.9g
- Carb: 5g
- Protein: 6.7g

Strawberry Bread

Prep time: 10 minutes
Cook time: 4 hours
Servings: 10 slices

Ingredients

- 5 eggs
- 1 egg white
- 1 ½ tsp. vanilla extract
- 2 tbsp. heavy whipping cream
- 2 tbsp. sour cream
- 1 cup monk fruit powder
- 1 ½ tsp. baking powder
- ½ tsp. salt
- ½ tsp. cinnamon
- 8 tbsp. butter, melted
- ¾ cup coconut flour
- ¾ cup chopped strawberries

Directions

1. Beat the eggs, egg white, vanilla, heavy cream, sour cream, baking powder, salt, and cinnamon until mixed.
2. Then stir in coconut flour and fold in strawberries until mixed.
3. Add the batter into the bread bucket and cover.
4. Select Basic/White cycle or low-carb. Press Start.
5. Remove the bread when done.
6. Cool, slice, and serve.

Nutritional Facts Per Serving

- Calories: 201
- Fat: 16.4g
- Carb: 6.1g
- Protein: 4.7g

Cranberry and Orange Bread

Prep time: 10 minutes
Cook time: 4 hours
Servings: 12

Ingredients
- 1 cup chopped cranberries
- ⅔ cup 3 tbsp. monk fruit powder, divided
- 5 eggs
- 1 egg white
- 2 tbsp. sour cream
- 1 ½ tsp. orange extract
- 1 tsp. vanilla extract
- 9 tbsp. butter, unsalted and melted
- 9 tbsp. coconut flour
- 1 ½ tsp. baking powder
- ¼ tsp. salt

Directions
1. Place cranberries in a bowl and stir in 3 tbsp. of monk fruit powder until combined. Set aside.
2. Crack eggs in a bowl. Beat in the remaining ingredients in it until mixed. Then fold in cranberries until just mixed.
3. Add batter into the bread bucket and cover.
4. Select Basic/White cycle or low-carb, then press Start.
5. Remove the bread when done.
6. Cool, slice, and serve.

Nutritional Facts Per Serving
- Calories: 149
- Fat: 13.1g
- Carb: 4g
- Protein: 3.9g

Blueberry Bread

<u>Prep time: 10 minutes</u>
<u>Cook time: 4 hours</u>
<u>Servings: 16 slices</u>

Ingredients
- 4 eggs
- 3 tbsp. heavy whipping cream
- 3 tbsp. butter, unsalted and melted
- 1 tsp. vanilla extract
- 2 tbsp. coconut flour
- 2 cups almond flour
- ½ cup erythritol sweetener
- 1 ½ tsp. baking powder
- 1 cup blueberries

Directions
1. Beat eggs, cream, butter, and vanilla until combined.
2. Place flours in a bowl. Then stir in sweetener and baking powder until mixed, and fold in blueberries.
3. Add egg mixture into the bread bucket and top with flour mixture. Cover.
4. Select Basic/White cycle or low-carb. Press Start.
5. Remove the bread when done.
6. Cool, slice, and serve.

Nutritional Facts Per Serving
- Calories: 211
- Fat: 18.2g
- Carb: 5.9g
- Protein: 7.7g

Chocolate Bread

Prep time: 10 minutes
Cook time: 4 hours
Servings: 8 slices

Ingredients
- 3 eggs
- ¼ cup Swerve sweetener
- ¼ cup melted coconut oil
- 2 tbsp. almond flour
- ¼ cup coconut flour
- ¼ tbsp. salt
- 2 tbsp. whey protein powder
- ½ tsp. baking soda
- ½ cup cocoa powder
- 2 tbsp. mini chocolate chips, sugar-free

Directions
1. Crack eggs in a bowl. Beat until frothy and then beat in Swerve sweetener and oil until fluffy.
2. Place flours in another bowl. Stir in remaining ingredients until mixed.
3. Add egg mixture into the bread bucket and top with flour mixture. Cover.
4. Select Basic/White cycle or low-carb. Press Start.
5. Remove the bread when done.
6. Cool, slice, and serve.

Nutritional Facts Per Serving
- Calories: 214
- Fat: 18g
- Carb: 3.7g
- Protein: 6.4g

Delicious Lemon Bread

Prep time: 10 minutes
Cook time: 3 hours and 25 minutes
Servings: 15

Ingredients
- 6 eggs
- 9 tbsp. melted butter
- 2 tbsp. softened cream cheese
- 1 tsp. vanilla
- 2 tbsp. heavy whipping cream
- ½ cup and 2 tbsp. coconut flour
- ½ tsp. salt
- 1 ½ tsp. baking powder
- ⅔ cup Monk fruit sweetener
- Zests of 2 lemons
- 4 tsp. fresh lemon juice

For the glaze
- 2 tbsp. powdered Monk fruit sweetener
- 2 tsp. fresh lemon juice
- 1 tsp. lemon zest
- A splash of heavy whipping cream

Directions
1. Add everything in the bread machine according to the order recommended by the machine manufacturer.
2. Select Sweet bread and press Start. Check the bread after 5 minutes to know its consistency.
3. Remove the bread when done and cool.
4. Mix all the glaze ingredients in a bowl and pour the glaze over the bread.
5. Slice and serve.

Nutritional Facts Per Serving
- Calories: 121
- Fat: 10g
- Carb: 3g
- Protein: 3g

Strawberry Bread

Prep time: 10 minutes
Cook time: 3 hours and 25 minutes
Servings: 12 slices

Ingredients
- 5 eggs
- 1 egg white
- 8 tbsp. of melted butter
- ½ tsp. of cinnamon
- 2 tbsp. of sour cream
- 1 cup of powdered Monk fruit
- 1 ½ tsp. of vanilla
- 2 tbsp. of heavy whipping cream
- 12 tbsp. of coconut flour
- ½ tsp. salt
- 1 ½ tsp. of baking powder
- 3/4 cup of chopped fresh strawberries

For the icing
- 3/4 cup of powdered Monk fruit
- 1 tbsp. of melted butter
- 2 tbsp. of heavy whipping cream
- ¼ cup of chopped fresh strawberries
- A dash of vanilla

Directions
1. Add eggs, egg white, butter, cinnamon, sour cream, sweetener, vanilla, whipping cream, flour, baking powder, and salt in the bread machine. Press Basic/White bread.
2. Check the dough after 10 minutes in the mixing process.
3. Add the rest of the ingredients after the beep.
4. Remove the bread when done.
5. Whisk all the glaze ingredients in a bowl.
6. Pour the icing over the bread.
7. Slice and serve.

Nutritional Facts Per Serving
- Calories: 192
- Fat: 16g
- Carb: 6g
- Protein: 4g

Delicious Pumpkin Bread

Prep time: 10 minutes
Cook time: 3 hours and 25 minutes
Servings: 12

Ingredients
- 1 cup of creamy unsweetened almond butter
- 2 large eggs
- ⅔ cup of erythritol
- ⅔ cup of canned pumpkin puree
- 1 tsp. of baking powder
- ½ tsp. of ground cinnamon
- ½ tsp. of ground nutmeg
- 1/8 tsp. of ground ginger
- 1/8 tsp. of ground garlic cloves

Directions
1. Add everything in the bread machine according to bread machine instructions.
2. Select Basic setting. Press Start.
3. Cool, slice, and serve.

Nutritional Facts Per Serving
- Calories: 143
- Fat: 12g
- Carb: 6g
- Protein: 6g

Delicious Cranberry and Cream Cheese

Prep time: 10 minutes
Cook time: 3 hours and 25 minutes
Servings: 10 slices

Ingredients
- ½ cup erythritol
- ½ cup unsalted and soft butter
- 8 oz. softened cream cheese
- 4 eggs
- 1 tsp. vanilla extract
- ½ cup of coconut flour
- ½ tsp. baking powder
- ½ tsp. salt
- 1 cup cranberries

Directions
1. Add in the sweetener, butter, cream cheese, eggs, vanilla extract, coconut flour, baking powder, and salt to taste in the bread machine.
2. Select Basic White and press Start.
3. Check the dough after 10 minutes. Add in the remaining ingredients after the beep.
4. Cool, slice, and serve.

Nutritional Facts Per Serving
- Calories: 153
- Fat: 13g
- Carb: 6g
- Protein: 4g

Chocolate Bread

Prep time: 10 minutes
Cook time: 3 hours and 25 minutes
Servings: 8 slices

Ingredients
- 6 large eggs
- ½ cup of Swerve
- ½ cup of unsalted butter
- ½ cup of coconut flour
- ¼ cup of almond flour
- ¼ cup of protein powder
- ½ tsp. of salt to taste
- 1 tsp. of baking soda
- ¼ cup of cocoa powder
- ¼ cup of chocolate chips

Directions
1. Add in the eggs, Swerve sweetener, butter, coconut flour, almond flour, protein powder, baking soda, cocoa powder, and salt to the taste.
2. Select Basic White and press start.
3. Check the dough after 10 minutes.
4. Add the rest of the ingredients after the beep.
5. Cool the bread, slice, and serve.

Nutritional Facts Per Serving
- Calories: 206
- Fat: 17g
- Carb: 6g
- Protein: 6g

Keto Apple Bread

Prep time: 10 minutes
Cook time: 3 hours and 25 minutes
Servings: 12

Ingredients
- 2 cups of almond flour
- ½ cup of ground flaxseed
- ½ cup of Swerve
- 2 tsp. cinnamon
- 3/4 tsp. salt to taste
- 3/4 tsp. baking soda
- ½ tsp. nutmeg
- 4 tbsp. coconut oil
- 4 large eggs
- ¼ cup of heavy cream or coconut cream
- ¼ cup of water
- 2 tsp. pure vanilla extract
- 1 ½ tsp. apple cider vinegar
- ½ tsp. blackstrap molasses
- ¼ tsp. Stevia glycerite
- 2 diced apples

Directions
1. Add in the flour, ground flaxseed, Swerve, cinnamon, baking soda, nutmeg, coconut oil, eggs, heavy cream, water, vanilla extract, vinegar, molasses, Stevia, and salt to the bread machine.
2. Select Basic White and press Start.
3. Check the dough after 10 minutes.
4. Add the rest of the ingredients once the machine beeps.
5. Cool, slice, and serve.

Nutritional Facts Per Serving
- Calories: 242
- Fat: 20g
- Carb: 11g
- Protein: 7g

Low-Carb Cranberry and Walnut Bread

Prep time: 10 minutes
Cook time: 3 hours and 25 minutes
Servings: 16

Ingredients
- 1 cup of blanched almond flour
- ¼ cup of coconut flour
- 3/4 cup of Swerve
- 2 ½ tsp. of baking powder
- 1 tsp. sea salt to taste
- 1 tsp. baking soda
- 1 tsp. ground cinnamon
- Zest of one orange
- Juice of one lemon
- 2 tbsp. coconut oil
- 2 eggs
- 1 ½ cups of fresh cranberries
- ½ cup of walnuts

Directions
1. Add in the almond flour, coconut flour, Swerve, baking powder, baking soda, cinnamon, orange zest, lemon juice, coconut oil, and eggs in the bread machine.
2. Select Basic White and press Start.
3. Check the dough after ten minutes.
4. Add the rest of the ingredients after the beep.
5. Remove the bread when done.
6. Cool, slice, and serve.

Nutritional Facts Per Serving
- Calories: 104
- Fat: 5g
- Carb: 5g
- Protein: 3g

Chocolate and Pistachio Bread

Prep time: 10 minutes
Cook time: 3 hours and 25 minutes
Servings: 24

Ingredients
- ⅔ cup of granulated keto sugar
- ½ cup of unsalted butter
- 1 cup of almond milk
- 2 eggs
- 1 ½ cups of almond flour
- 1 cup of chopped and roasted pistachio nuts
- ½ cup of chocolate chips
- ⅓ cup of unsweetened baking cocoa
- 1 ½ tsp. of baking powder
- ¼ tsp. of salt to taste

Directions
1. Add in the flour, granulated sugar, butter, almond milk, eggs, baking cocoa, baking powder, and salt to the bread machine.
2. Select Basic White and press Start.
3. Check the dough after 10 minutes.
4. Add the rest of the ingredients after the beep.
5. Remove the bread when done.
6. Cool, slice, and serve.

Nutritional Facts Per Serving
- Calories: 133
- Fat: 8g
- Carb: 10g
- Protein: 3g

Low-Carb Date and Walnut Bread

Prep time: 10 minutes
Cook time: 3 hours and 25 minutes
Servings: 8 slices

Ingredients
- ½ cup of blanched almond flour
- 2 tbsp. of coconut flour
- 1/8 tsp. of sea salt to taste
- ¼ tsp. of baking soda
- 3 large dates with the pits removed
- 3 large eggs
- 1 tbsp. of apple cider vinegar
- ½ cup of chopped walnuts

Directions
1. Add in the almond flour, coconut flour, baking soda, eggs, vinegar, and salt to the bread machine.
2. Select Basic Bread and press Start.
3. Check the dough after 10 minutes.
4. Add the rest of the ingredients after the machine beeps.
5. Remove the bread when done.
6. Cool, slice, and serve.

Nutritional Facts Per Serving
- Calories: 147
- Fat: 7g
- Carb: 9g
- Protein: 4g

Buttermilk Bread

Prep time: 10 minutes
Cook time: 3 hours and 25 minutes
Servings: 16

Ingredients
- 17.6 oz. of buttermilk
- 2 eggs
- 4.6 oz. of linseed flour
- 1.4 oz. of almond flour
- 1.4 oz. of psyllium husks
- 2 oz. chia seeds
- 0.7 oz. of sunflower seed flour
- 1 tsp. of baking soda
- 1 tsp. of salt to taste

Directions
1. Add everything in the bread machine according to bread machine recommendation.
2. Select Basic/White bread setting.
3. Check the dough after ten minutes.
4. Cool, slice, and serve.

Nutritional Facts Per Serving
- Calories: 155
- Fat: 6.8g
- Carb: 8.3g
- Protein: 11.5g

Peach Cake Bread

Prep time: 10 minutes
Cook time: 3 hours and 25 minutes
Servings: 12

Ingredients
- 3 tsp. softened butter
- ½ cup of erythritol
- 1 cup of almond flour
- 1 cup of coconut flour
- ½ tsp. salt to taste
- 2 tsp. baking powder
- ¼ tsp. allspice
- 1/8 tsp. ground nutmeg
- 1 tsp. ground cinnamon
- 2 eggs
- 3/4 cup of olive oil
- ¼ cup of almond milk
- 1 ½ cups of peeled and diced peaches

Directions
1. Add in all the ingredients except for the peaches.
2. Select Basic bread setting and press Start.
3. Check the dough after ten minutes.
4. Add the diced peaches after the beep.
5. Cool, slice, and serve.

Nutritional Facts Per Serving
- Calories: 154
- Fat: 14.5g
- Carb: 3.8g
- Protein: 3.5g

Garlic and Dill Bread

Prep time: 10 minutes
Cook time: 3 hours and 25 minutes
Servings: 10 slices

Ingredients
- 1 ½ cups almond flour
- 4 large eggs
- 1 scoop of egg white protein
- 5 tbsp. of unsalted butter
- ¼ tsp. of kosher salt to taste
- 4 tsp. of baking powder
- ¼ tsp. of cream of tartar
- 1 tsp. of garlic powder
- ¼ tbsp. of dried dill weed
- 8 oz. of cheddar cheese

Directions
1. Add in the flour, eggs, egg white protein, butter, baking powder, cream of tartar, garlic powder, dried dill, cheese, and salt to the bread machine.
2. Select White bread and press Start.
3. Check the dough after five minutes.
4. Remove the bread when done.
5. Cool, slice, and serve.

Nutritional Facts Per Serving
- Calories: 288
- Fat: 10g
- Carb: 4g
- Protein: 14g

Chocolate, Mixed Berry, and Nuts Bread

Prep time: 10 minutes
Cook time: 3 hours and 25 minutes
Servings: 10 slices

Ingredients
- ½ cup of coconut flour
- 5 eggs
- ½ cup of erythritol
- ½ cup of unsalted butter
- ¼ tsp. salt to taste
- ½ tsp. of vanilla extract
- 3 tbsp. of coconut milk
- 1 cup of mixed berries of choice
- ⅓ cup of chopped pecans, walnuts, or almonds as desired
- ¼ cup of cocoa powder

Directions
1. Add in flour, eggs, sweetener, butter, vanilla extract, coconut milk, cocoa powder, and salt.
2. Select Basic bread setting. Press Start.
3. Check the dough after 10 minutes.
4. Add the remaining ingredients after the beep.
5. Cool, slice, and serve.

Nutritional Facts Per Serving
- Calories: 165
- Fat: 14g
- Carb: 7g
- Protein: 4g

Low-Carb Wheat-Style Bread

Prep time: 10 minutes
Cook time: 3 hours and 25 minutes
Servings: 14

Ingredients
- ½ cups of almond flour
- ⅓ cups of ground flaxseed
- ¼ cups of whole psyllium husks
- ½ tsp. of cinnamon
- ½ tsp. pink salt to taste
- 2 ½ tsp. baking powder
- ½ tbsp. Swerve
- ¼ cups of water
- 2 tbsp. olive oil
- 4 large eggs
- 1 ½ tbsp. of apple cider vinegar
- 2 ½ tbsp. of hemp hearts
- ¼ tsp. of baking soda

Directions
1. Add in the ground flaxseed, almond flour, psyllium husks, cinnamon, baking powder, sweetener, water, oil, eggs, vinegar, hemp hearts, baking soda, and salt to the bread machine.
2. Select White bread setting and press Start.
3. Check the dough after ten minutes.
4. Cool, slice, and serve.

Nutritional Facts Per Serving
- Calories: 84
- Fat: 6.4g
- Carb: 3.5g
- Protein: 3.1g

Lemon and Blueberry Bread

Prep time: 10 minutes
Cook time: 3 hours 25 minutes
Servings: 10 slices

Ingredients
- 2 cups of almond flour
- 2 tsp. of baking powder
- ½ lemon zest
- ½ cup of erythritol
- 2 eggs
- 1 cup of heavy whipping cream
- ¼ cup of melted butter
- 1 tbsp. of lemon juice
- 1 cup of blueberries

Directions
1. Add in the almond flour, baking powder, lemon zest, sweetener, eggs, whipping cream, melted butter, and lemon juice in the bread machine.
2. Select White/basic bread setting. Press Start.
3. Check the dough after ten minutes.
4. Add the remaining ingredients after the machine beeps.
5. Remove the bread when done.
6. Cool, slice, and serve.

Nutritional Facts Per Serving
- Calories: 267
- Fat: 25g
- Carb: 7g
- Protein: 6g

Orange Bread

Prep time: 10 minutes
Cook time: 3 hours 25 minutes
Servings: 16

Ingredients
- 3 cups of almond flour
- ⅓ cup of unflavored whey protein powder
- 1 ½ tsp. of baking powder
- 1 tsp. of baking soda
- ½ tsp. salt to taste
- ½ cup of softened butter
- ½ cup of granulated Swerve
- 3 large eggs
- Zest of a medium orange
- 20 drops of stevia extract
- ¼ cup of orange juice
- ¼ cup of almond milk

Chocolate glaze
- 2 oz. of melted chocolate
- 2 tbsp. of melted butter
- 2 tbsp. of powdered Swerve
- ½ tsp. of vanilla extract

Directions
1. Add the bread ingredients to the bread machine.
2. Select Basic/white bread and press Start.
3. Check the dough after ten minutes.
4. Remove the bread when done.
5. Whisk the glaze ingredients in a bowl.
6. Pour over the bread. Slice and serve it.

Nutritional Facts Per Serving
- Calories: 198
- Fat: 16g
- Carb: 6.6g
- Protein: 18g

Low-Carb Pound Cake Loaf

Prep time: 10 minutes
Cook time: 3 hours and 25 minutes
Servings: 10

Ingredients for pound cake
- 2 ½ cups of almond flour
- ½ cup of unsalted and softened butter
- 1 ½ cups of erythritol
- 8 eggs
- 1 ½ tsp. of vanilla extract
- ½ tsp. lemon extract
- ½ tsp. salt
- 8 oz. cream cheese
- 1 ½ tsp. of baking powder

Glaze
- ¼ cup of powdered erythritol
- 3 tbsp. heavy whipping cream
- ½ tsp. of vanilla extract

Directions
1. Add everything in the bread machine according to bread machine recommendation.
2. Select Basic bread setting and press Start.
3. Check the dough after 10 minutes.
4. Remove the bread when done.
5. Whisk the glaze ingredients in a bowl.
6. Pour over the bread. Slice and serve the bread.

Nutritional Facts Per Serving
- Calories: 254
- Fat: 23.4g
- Carb: 2.49g
- Protein: 7.9g

Red Velvet Cake

Prep time: 10 minutes
Cook time: 1 hour 30 minutes
Servings: 10 slices

Ingredients
- ½ cup of unsalted butter
- ¼ cup of powdered erythritol
- 2 eggs
- 1 cup of sour cream
- 1 ½ cup of almond flour
- ¼ cup of coconut flour
- 2 tbsp. cocoa powder
- 1 tbsp. of apple cider vinegar
- 1 ½ tsp. of baking soda
- 1 oz. of red food coloring plus 1 tbsp. of coconut flour mixed together
- 1 tsp. of vanilla
- 1 ½ tsp. of red velvet emulsion

Frosting
- 8 oz. of cream cheese
- 4 tbsp. of butter
- ¼ cup of heavy cream
- 2 tbsp. of erythritol sweetener

Directions
1. Add everything in the bread machine according to bread machine recommendation.
2. Select the Cake cycle and press Start.
3. Once the kneading process goes halfway, scrap down the sides of the baking pan with a spatula, then bake as directed until fully baked.
4. Remove the cake when done.
5. Mix a bowl, add in the cream cheese and butter, then mix to combine. Add in the sweetener, and the heavy cream, then mix everything together to combine. Frost the cake and serve.

Nutritional Facts Per Serving
- Calories: 357
- Fat: 33g
- Carb: 8g
- Protein: 8g

Vegan Keto Bread

Prep time: 10 minutes
Cook time: 3 hours and 25 minutes
Servings: 16

Ingredients
- 1 cup of almond flour
- 1 cup of pumpkin flour
- ½ cup of coconut flour
- ⅓ cup of ground psyllium husk
- ¼ cup of chia seeds
- 1 tbsp. of baking powder
- 1 tsp. salt to taste
- 2 tbsp. olive oil
- 1 tsp. of apple cider vinegar
- 2 cups of warm water

Directions
1. Add everything in the bread machine according to bread machine recommendation.
2. Select Basic bread setting and press Start.
3. Check the dough after ten minutes.
4. Remove the bread when done.
5. Cool, slice, and serve.

Nutritional Facts Per Serving
- Calories: 117
- Fat: 7.8g
- Carb: 4.3g
- Protein: 3.9g

Zucchini Bread

Prep time: 10 minutes
Cook time: 3 hours and 25 minutes
Servings: 8 slices

Ingredients
- 2 cups of almond flour
- ½ tsp. kosher salt to taste
- ½ tsp. ground cinnamon
- ½ cup Swerve sweetener
- 1 tsp. baking soda
- 2 beaten eggs
- ¼ cup of melted butter
- 1 ½ cups of grated zucchini

Directions
1. Add everything in the bread machine according to bread machine instructions. Select the Basic bread.
2. Once the kneading process goes halfway, scrap down the sides of the baking pan with a spatula.
3. Remove the bread when done.
4. Cool, slice, and serve.

Nutritional Facts Per Serving
- Calories: 249
- Fat: 22g
- Carb: 7g
- Protein: 8g

Raspberry Bread

Prep time: 10 minutes
Cook time: 50 minutes
Servings: 12 slices

Ingredients
- 1 cup raspberries
- ¼ cup favorite sugar substitute
- 1 ½ tsp. keto baking powder
- 2 cups almond flour
- 4 tbsp. sour cream
- 4 tbsp. unsalted butter, melted
- 2 whole eggs
- 1 tsp. vanilla
- 1 tsp. lemon extract
- ½ lemon, juiced

Directions
1. Add everything in the bread machine except the raspberries.
2. Cover and select Cake. Add the raspberries after the beep.
3. Press Start.
4. Remove the bread when done.
5. Cool, slice, and serve.

Nutritional Facts Per Serving
- Calories: 168
- Fat: 14.8g
- Carb: 8.3g
- Protein: 5.3g

Blueberry Bread

Prep time: 10 minutes
Cook time: 50 minutes
Servings: 12 slices

Ingredients
- ½ cup blueberries
- ⅓ cup of your favorite sugar substitute
- 2 tsp. keto baking powder
- 2 cups almond flour
- 4 tbsp. sour cream
- 4 tbsp. unsalted butter, melted
- 2 whole eggs
- 1 tsp. vanilla

Directions
1. Beat eggs and pour them into the bread machine. Add all the other ingredients except the blueberries.
2. Close and press Cake.
3. Add the blueberries after the beep.
4. Remove the bread when done.
5. Cool, slice, and serve.

Nutritional Facts Per Serving
- Calories: 165
- Fat: 14.8g
- Carb: 9.8g
- Protein: 5.1g

Chocolate Bread

Prep time: 10 minutes
Cook time: 50 to 70 minutes
Servings: 12

Ingredients
- 6 whole eggs, well-beaten
- ½ tsp. vanilla
- ½ tsp. Stevia
- 2 tsp. apple cider vinegar
- 4 oz. salted butter, melted
- 1 oz. unsweetened baking chocolate, melted
- ¾ cups coconut flour
- ½ cup your favorite keto sweetener
- ¼ cup unsweetened cocoa powder
- 1 tsp. keto baking powder
- ½ tsp. baking soda
- ½ tsp. instant keto coffee
- ½ tsp. sea salt
- ¼ tsp. xanthan gum
- 2 tbsp. sugar-free chocolate chips (for garnish)

Directions
1. Mix all the dry ingredients in a bowl.
2. In a small bowl, beat the eggs.
3. Pour eggs and add all of the wet ingredients into the bread machine pan.
4. Cover them with the dry ingredients.
5. Close the cover.
6. Select Cake and press Start.
7. Remove the bread when done.
8. Decorate the bread with chocolate chips if desired. Cool, slice, and serve.

Nutritional Facts Per Serving
- Calories: 129
- Fat: 12g
- Carb: 8g
- Protein: 3.8g

Banana Bread

Prep time: 10 minutes
Cook time: 60 to 70 minutes
Servings: 16

Ingredients
- 2½ cup almond flour
- 1 cup mashed banana
- 6 large organic eggs, beaten
- 4 tbsp. ghee, melted
- ½ cup erythritol
- 2 tbsp. cinnamon
- 1 tbsp. keto baking powder
- ½ cup walnuts, crushed
- ¼ tsp. ground nutmeg

Directions
1. Mix all the dry ingredients in a bowl.
2. Beat the eggs in a bowl. Pour eggs and all of the wet ingredients into the bread machine pan.
3. Cover them with the dry ingredients.
4. Close. Press Dough and start.
5. Once the process completes, start the Bake mode for 55 minutes.
6. Remove the bread when done.
7. Cool, slice, and serve.

Nutritional Facts Per Serving
- Calories: 191
- Fat: 16.2g
- Carb: 11.9g
- Protein: 7.2g

Avocado Bread

Prep time: 10 minutes
Cook time: 60 to 70 minutes
Servings: 14 slices

Ingredients
- 4 avocados, mashed
- 2 cups almond flour
- 1 cup coconut flour
- ½ cup Monk fruit sweetener
- 5 tbsp. avocado oil
- 4 tbsp. unsweetened cocoa powder
- ½ tsp. kosher salt
- 1 tsp. baking soda
- 1 tsp. vanilla extract
- 1 cup of chocolate chips

Directions
1. Mix all the dry ingredients in a bowl.
2. Combine all the wet ingredients in a blender.
3. Pour all of the wet ingredients into the bread machine pan.
4. Cover them with the dry ingredients. Add half of the chocolate chips.
5. Close and select Cake. Press Start.
6. Allow the machine to knead.
7. Before the baking, top the bread with the remaining ½ cup of chocolate chips.
8. Remove the bread when done.
9. Cool, slice, and serve.

Nutritional Facts Per Serving
- Calories: 290
- Fat: 24.1g
- Carb: 10.7g
- Protein: 5.9g

Gingerbread Cake

Prep time: 10 minutes
Cook time: 45 minutes
Servings: 10 slices

Ingredients
- 4 large organic eggs
- ¼ cup unsalted organic butter, melted
- 1 tsp. vanilla extract
- ¾ cup granulated Swerve
- ¾ cup coconut flour
- 1 tsp. keto baking powder
- 2 tsp. ground ginger
- 2 tsp. ground cinnamon
- ½ tsp. ground allspice
- ½ tsp. ground nutmeg
- ½ tsp. ground cloves
- ¼ tsp. kosher salt

For Icing
- ½ cup cream cheese, softened
- ¼ cup Swerve, powdered
- 1 tsp. vanilla extract
- ¼ cup walnuts, chopped

Directions
1. Whisk together the eggs, vanilla, and unsalted butter.
2. Mix all the dry ingredients in a large bowl.
3. Pour all the wet ingredients into the bread machine pan.
4. Cover them with the dry ingredients.
5. Close and press Cake.
6. Remove the cake when done.
7. Combine cream cheese, vanilla extract, and sweetener. Cover the bread and sprinkle with nuts.
8. Cool, slice, and serve.

Nutritional Facts Per Serving
- Calories: 140
- Fat: 12.9g
- Carb: 9g
- Protein: 4.4g

Lemon Bread

Prep time: 10 minutes
Cook time: 1 hour
Servings: 12

Ingredients
- 9.5 oz. almond flour
- ½ tsp. keto baking powder
- ½ cup erythritol
- 2 tbsp. poppy seeds
- Zest of 2 lemons
- 2 tbsp. lemon juice
- 3 tbsp. unsalted butter, melted
- 6 whole eggs

For icing
- ½ cup powdered erythritol
- 1 tbsp. lemon juice
- 2 tbsp. water

Directions
1. Put all ingredients into the bread machine pan.
2. Close the cover.
3. Select Cake and press Start.
4. Remove the bread when done.
5. Make the icing in a small bowl.
6. Drizzle it over the bread.
7. Cool, slice, and serve.

Nutritional Facts Per Serving
- Calories: 193
- Fat: 17g
- Carb: 8g
- Protein: 7.9g

Holiday Bread

Prep time: 10 minutes
Cook time: 1 hour
Servings: 12 slices

Ingredients
- 2½ cups almond flour
- 2 cups whey isolate
- 1 cup lukewarm water
- ¼ cup almond milk
- ½ cup powdered erythritol
- ½ cup butter, melted
- 1½ tbsp. keto baking powder
- 2 tsp. xanthan gum
- ½ tsp. sea salt

For icing
- ½ cup powdered erythritol
- 1 tbsp. lemon juice
- 2 tbsp. water

Directions
1. Put all ingredients into the bread machine pan.
2. Close and press Cake. Press Start.
3. Remove the bread when done.
4. Mix the icing ingredients in a bowl.
5. Drizzle it over the bread.
6. Cool, slice, and serve.

Nutritional Facts Per Serving
- Calories: 130
- Fat: 11.8g
- Carb: 5g
- Protein: 5.3g

American Cheese Beer Bread

Prep time: 10 minutes
Cook time: 3 hours and 25 minutes
Servings: 10

Ingredients
- 1 ½ cups of almond flour
- 3 tsp. unsalted melted butter
- 1 tsp. salt
- 1 egg
- 2 tsp. Swerve sweetener
- 1 cup, Keto low-carb beer
- ¾ tsp. baking powder
- ½ tsp. cheddar cheese, shredded
- ½ tsp. active dry yeast

Directions
1. In a bowl, mix almond flour, Swerve sweetener, salt, shredded cheddar cheese, and baking powder.
2. In another bowl, mix butter, egg, and beer.
3. Add everything, including the yeast, in the bread machine, according to bread machine recommendation.
4. Cover and select Basic bread.
5. Remove the bread when done.
6. Cool, slice, and serve.

Nutritional Facts Per Serving
- Calories: 94
- Fat: 6g
- Carb: 4g
- Protein: 1g

Date and Walnut Bread

Prep time: 10 minutes
Cook time: 3 hours and 25 minutes
Servings: 8

Ingredients
- ½ cup almond flour
- 2 tbsp. coconut flour
- 1/8 tsp. sea salt
- ¼ tsp. baking soda
- 3 large dates with pits removed
- 3 eggs
- 1 tbsp. apple cider vinegar
- ½ cup chopped walnuts

Directions
1. Add everything in the bread machine except nuts and fruits.
2. Select Fruit bread and press Start.
3. Add the nuts and fruits after the beep.
4. Remove the bread when done.
5. Cool, slice, and serve.

Nutritional Facts Per Serving
- Calories: 147
- Fat: 7g
- Carb: 9g
- Protein: 4g

CHAPTER 6. MORE BREAD RECIPES

Basil Cheese Bread

Prep time: 10 minutes
Cook time: 3 hours 25 minutes
Servings: 10 slices

Ingredients
- 2 cups almond flour
- 1 cup warm water
- ½ tsp. salt
- 1 tsp. dried basil
- ½ cup of shredded mozzarella cheese
- ¼ tsp. active dry yeast
- 3 tsp. melted unsalted butter
- 1 tsp. Stevia powder

Directions
1. In a bowl, combine the almond flour, dried basil, salt, shredded mozzarella cheese, and stevia powder.
2. Combine warm water and melted unsalted butter in another bowl.
3. Add everything in the bread machine pan, including the yeast, according to bread machine recommendation.
4. Select Sweet bread setting and press Start.
5. Remove the bread when done.
6. Cool, slice, and serve.

Nutritional Facts Per Serving
- Calories: 124
- Fat: 8g
- Carb: 8g
- Protein: 11g

Cheese Sausage Bread

Prep time: 10 minutes
Cook time: 3 hours and 25 minutes
Servings: 8

Ingredients
- 1 tsp. dry yeast
- 3 ½ cups almond flour
- 1 tsp. salt
- 1 tbsp. granulated sugar
- 1 ½ tbsp. oil
- 2 tbsp. smoked sausage, chopped
- 2 tbsp. grated cheese
- 1 tbsp. chopped garlic
- 1 cup water

Directions
1. Add all the ingredients according to the directions.
2. Select Basic and press Start.
3. Remove the bread when done.
4. Cool, slice, and serve.

Nutritional Facts Per Serving
- Calories: 160
- Fat: 5.6g
- Carb: 4g
- Protein: 7.7g

French Ham Bread

Prep time: 10 minutes
Cook time: 3 hours 30 minutes
Servings: 8

Ingredients
- 3 ⅓ cups almond flour
- 1 cup ham, cubed
- ½ cup milk powder
- 1 ½ tbsp. granulated sugar
- 1 tsp. fresh yeast
- 1 tsp. salt
- 1 tsp. dried basil
- 1 ⅓ cups water
- 2 tbsp. olive oil

Directions
1. Put all the ingredients according to the directions of your bread maker.
2. Select Basic and press Start.
3. Remove the bread when done.
4. Cool, slice, and serve.

Nutritional Facts Per Serving
- Calories: 287
- Fat: 5.5g
- Carb: 2g
- Protein: 11.4g

Keto Onion Bread

Prep time: 10 minutes
Cook time: 3 hours 25 minutes
Servings: 12

Ingredients
- 1 ½ cups water
- 2 tbsp. + 2 tsp butter, unsalted
- 1 ½ tsp. salt
- 1 tbsp. + 1 tsp. granulated sugar
- 2 tbsp. + 2 tsp. almond milk
- 4 cups almond flour
- 2 tsp. active dry yeast
- 4 tbsp. dry onion soup mix

Directions
1. Add all ingredients except dry onion mix in the bread machine pan according to bread machine recommendation.
2. Select Basic cycle and then press Start.
3. Add the dry onion soup mix after the beep.
4. Remove the bread when done.
5. Cool, slice, and serve.

Nutritional Facts Per Serving
- Calories: 128
- Fat: 15.9g
- Carb: 4g
- Protein: 6.4g

Tomato Bread

Prep time: 10 minutes
Cook time: 45 minutes
Servings: 16

Ingredients
- 4 whole eggs
- 2 tbsp. salted butter, melted
- 1 cup flaxseed meal
- 2 tsp. keto baking powder
- 1½ tsp. xanthan gum
- ¼ tsp sea salt
- ½ tsp. dried basil
- ¼ tsp. garlic powder
- 2 tbsp. sun-dried tomatoes, diced
- ¼ cup parmesan, grated

Directions
1. Whisk eggs and butter together.
2. Pour all the ingredients into the bread machine pan.
3. Close and select Cake. Press Start.
4. Remove the bread when done.
5. Cool, slice, and serve.

Nutritional Facts Per Serving
- Calories: 88
- Fat: 6.1g
- Carb: 4g
- Protein: 4.7g

Keto Basil Parmesan Slices

Prep time: 10 minutes
Cook time: 3 hours and 25 minutes
Servings: 16

Ingredients
- 1 cup water
- ½ cup parmesan cheese, grated
- 3 tbsp. granulated sugar
- 1 tbsp. dried basil
- 1 ½ tbsp. olive oil
- 1 tsp. salt
- 3 cups almond flour
- 2 tsp. active dry yeast

Directions
1. Place everything in the bread machine pan according to bread machine recommendation.
2. Select Basic and press Start.
3. Remove the bread when done.
4. Cool, slice, and serve.

Nutritional Facts Per Serving
- Calories: 56
- Fat: 4.6g
- Carb: 4.3g
- Protein: 2.5g

Zucchini Bread

Prep time: 10 minutes
Cook time: 1 hour
Servings: 16

Ingredients
- 3 large whole eggs, slightly beaten
- ½ cup extra virgin olive oil
- 1 cup zucchini, grated
- 1 tsp. vanilla extract
- 2½ cup almond flour
- 1½ cup erythritol
- ½ tsp sea salt
- 1 tsp. cream of tartar
- ½ tsp. baking soda
- ½ tsp. nutmeg
- 1 tsp. ground cinnamon
- ¼ tsp. ground ginger
- ½ cup walnuts, chopped

Directions
1. Mix the cream of tartar with baking soda.
2. Combine all the dry ingredients in a bowl.
3. In another bowl, blend the wet ingredients and add the zucchini to this bowl.
4. Put everything in the bread machine and cover.
5. Choose Cake and press Start.
6. Add the walnuts after the beep.
7. Remove the bread when done.
8. Cool, slice, and serve.

Nutritional Facts Per Serving
- Calories: 171
- Fat: 16g
- Carb: 3.9g
- Protein: 6g

Bacon Bread

Prep time: 10 minutes
Cook time: 60 to 90 minutes
Servings: 12 slices

Ingredients
- 7 oz. bacon, diced and fried
- ⅓ cup sour cream, room temperature
- 2 whole eggs, room temperature
- 4 tbsp. salted butter, melted
- 1½ cup almond flour
- 1 tbsp. keto baking powder
- 1 cup parmesan, grated

Directions
1. Combine all the dry ingredients in a bowl.
2. Carefully whisk sour cream with eggs.
3. Pour all the ingredients into the bread machine pan.
4. Close and select Cake. Press Start.
5. Sprinkle cheese after the beep.
6. Remove the bread when done.
7. Cool, slice, and serve.

Nutritional Facts Per Serving
- Calories: 256
- Fat: 21.6g
- Carb: 2.6g
- Protein: 12.8g

Cauliflower Bread

Prep time: 10 minutes
Cook time: 75 minutes
Servings: 12 slices

Ingredients
- 3 cups cauliflower, cooked and mashed
- 6 egg whites, beaten
- 6 egg yolks
- 6 tbsp. avocado oil
- 1¼ cup almond flour
- 1 tbsp. keto baking powder
- 1 tsp. sea salt

Directions
1. Beat egg whites until peaks form.
2. Combine all of the dry ingredients in a bowl.
3. Pour all ingredients into the bread machine pan.
4. Close and select Cake. Press Start.
5. Remove the bread when done.
6. Cool, slice, and serve.

Nutritional Facts Per Serving
- Calories: 119
- Fat: 9.1g
- Carb: 2.7g
- Protein: 6.2g

Herb Bread

Prep time: 10 minutes
Cook time: 1 hour 10 minutes
Servings: 18 slices

Ingredients
- ½ cup warm water (90 °F)
- 4 whole eggs
- ¼ cup extra virgin olive oil
- 1 tbsp. olive tapenade (optional)
- 1 tsp. gluten-free baking powder
- 2 cups almond flour
- ¼ cup Psyllium husk powder
- 1 tsp sea salt
- 1 tbsp. sage
- 1 tbsp. dried oregano
- 1 tbsp. dried rosemary

Directions
1. Mix all the dry ingredients in a bowl.
2. Separate the eggs into whites and yolks. Whisk the whites until peaks form.
3. Add the wet ingredients into the dry mixture.
4. Combine and pour the bread batter into the bread machine pan.
5. Close and Select Quick Bread. Press Start.
6. Remove the bread when done.
7. Cool, slice, and serve.

Nutritional Facts Per Serving
- Calories: 119
- Fat: 10.2g
- Carb: 1.9g
- Protein: 4g

Cream Cheese Bread

Prep time: 10 minutes
Cook time: 1 hour 30 minutes
Servings: 12 slices

Ingredients
- 8 whole eggs, room temperature
- 8 oz. cream cheese, room temperature
- ½ cup unsalted butter, softened
- ½ cup sour cream, room temperature
- 1½ cups coconut flour
- 4 tsp. keto baking powder
- ½ tsp. Italian herbs
- 1 tsp. sea salt
- 1 tbsp. allulose
- 2 tbsp. sesame seeds, for garnish

Directions
1. Combine all the dry ingredients in a bowl, except the sesame seeds.
2. Carefully blend cream cheese with butter until fluffy. Add eggs to the mixture and combine.
3. Pour all the ingredients into the bread machine pan.
4. Close and select Cake. Press Start.
5. Remove the bread when done.
6. Cool, slice, and serve.

Nutritional Facts Per Serving
- Calories: 214
- Fat: 20.2g
- Carb: 3g
- Protein: 6g

Garlic Bread

Prep time: 10 minutes
Cook time: 50 minutes
Servings: 8 slices

Ingredients
- 2 cups almond flour
- 1 tsp. sea salt
- 1 tbsp. keto baking powder
- 1 tsp. garlic powder
- 1 whole egg, beaten
- ½ cup mozzarella cheese, shredded

For the Topping
- 1 tbsp. unsalted butter, melted
- ¼ tsp. garlic powder
- ¼ tsp. sea salt
- ¾ cup mozzarella cheese, shredded
- ½ tsp. rosemary

Directions
1. Put all the ingredients in the bread machine pan and cover.
2. Select Cake and press Start.
3. Remove the bread when done.
4. In a bowl, mix the melted butter, salt, and garlic powder.
5. Five minutes before the end of the baking process, brush the top of the bread with the garlic butter, then sprinkle with the shredded mozzarella cheese and rosemary.
6. Remove the bread when done.
7. Cool, slice, and serve.

Nutritional Facts Per Serving
- Calories: 176
- Fat: 14.9g
- Carb: 3.7g
- Protein: 7.3g

Sesame Bread

Prep time: 10 minutes
Cook time: 1 hour and 10 minutes
Servings: 18 slices

Ingredients
- ½ cup warm water (90 °F)
- 4 whole eggs
- ¼ cup sesame oil
- 1 tsp. gluten-free baking powder
- 2 cups almond flour
- ¼ cup Psyllium husk powder
- ½ tsp sea salt
- 1 tbsp. sesame seeds
- 1 tbsp. sunflower seeds

Directions
1. Combine all the dry ingredients in a bowl.
2. Separate the eggs into whites and yolks. Whisk the whites until peaks form.
3. Add the wet ingredients to the dry ingredients and carefully combine.
4. Pour the bread batter into the bread machine pan.
5. Close and select Quick Bread. Press Start.
6. Remove the bread when done.
7. Cool, slice, and serve.

Nutritional Facts Per Serving
- Calories: 123
- Fat: 10.6g
- Carb: 1.7g
- Protein: 4g

Scandinavian Bread

Prep time: 10 minutes
Cook time: 35 minutes
Servings: 12 slices

Ingredients
- 2½ cups almond flour
- 2 cups protein isolate
- 1 tbsp. xanthan gum
- 1 tbsp. pumpkin seeds
- 1 tbsp. hemp hearts
- 1 tbsp. chia seeds
- 3 tsp. keto baking powder
- ½ tsp. sea salt
- 1 cup warm water (90 °F)
- 2 tbsp. avocado oil

Directions
1. Add all the ingredients to the bread machine pan according to recommendation and cover.
2. Select Cake and press Start.
3. Remove the bread when done.
4. Cool, slice, and serve.

Nutritional Facts Per Serving
- Calories: 206
- Fat: 13.9g
- Carb: 3.2g
- Protein: 17.3g

Feta Oregano Bread

Prep time: 10 minutes
Cook time: 3 hours and 25 minutes
Servings: 10

Ingredients
- 1 cup almond flour
- 1 cup crumbled feta cheese
- ½ cup warm water
- 1 tsp. dried oregano
- ⅔ tsp. baking powder
- 1 tsp. extra virgin olive oil
- ½ tsp. salt
- 1 tsp. Swerve sweetener
- ¼ tsp. garlic powder
- 1 tsp. dried active yeast

Directions
1. In a bowl, add almond flour, Swerve sweetener, cheese, dried oregano, baking powder, garlic, and salt.
2. Combine the oil and warm water in another bowl.
3. Add everything in the bread machine, including the yeast, and cover.
4. Select Sweet bread and press Start.
5. Remove the bread when done.
6. Cool, slice, and serve.

Nutritional Facts Per Serving
- Calories: 114
- Fat: 7g
- Carb: 8g
- Protein: 9g

Cottage Cheese Bread

Prep time: 10 minutes
Cook time: 3 hours and 25 minutes
Servings: 12

Ingredients
- ½ cup water
- 1 cup cottage cheese
- 2 tbsp. margarine
- 1 egg
- 1 tbsp. granulated sugar
- ¼ tsp baking soda
- 1 tsp salt
- 3 cups almond flour
- 2 ½ tsp active dry yeast

Directions
1. Add everything to the bread machine.
2. Select Basic bread and press Start.
3. Remove the bread when done.
4. Cool, slice, and serve.

Nutritional Facts Per Serving
- Calories: 171
- Fat: 3.6g
- Carb: 6g
- Protein: 7.3g

Parmesan Cheddar Bread

Prep time: 10 minutes
Cook time: 3 hours and 25 minutes
Servings: 10

Ingredients
- 1 cup parmesan cheese, grated
- 1 cup almond flour
- ½ tsp. baking powder
- ¾ tsp. salt
- ¼ tsp. cayenne pepper
- ½ cup unsweetened almond milk
- ⅓ cup sour cream
- 1 tsp. active dry yeast
- 2 tsp. unsalted melted butter
- 1 egg

Directions
1. Mix almond flour, parmesan cheese, cayenne pepper, baking powder, and salt in a bowl.
2. In another bowl, combine the almond milk, sour cream, egg, and butter.
3. Pour the ingredients, including the yeast, in the bread machine according to bread machine recommendation.
4. Select Basic bread and press Start.
5. Remove the bread when done.
6. Cool, slice, and serve.

Nutritional Facts Per Serving
- Calories: 134
- Fat: 6.8g
- Carb: 4.2g
- Protein: 12.1g

Pepper Cheddar Bread

Prep time: 10 minutes
Cook time: 3 hours 25 minutes
Servings: 10

Ingredients
- ½ cup coconut flour
- 1 cup almond flour
- 1 tsp. black pepper powder
- ¾ cup warm water
- 1 cup cheddar cheese, grated
- 1 tsp. salt
- 2 tsp. unsalted melted butter
- 1 tsp. baking powder
- 1 tsp. active dry yeast

Directions
1. In a bowl, combine the almond flour, coconut flour, shredded cheddar cheese, black pepper powder, baking powder, and salt.
2. Combine the warm water and unsalted melted butter.
3. Add everything in the bread machine, including yeast, according to bread machine recommendation.
4. Select Basic bread and press Start.
5. Cool, slice, and serve.

Nutritional Facts Per Serving
- Calories: 84
- Fat: 4g
- Carb: 3g
- Protein: 1g

Olive Cheese Bread

Prep time: 10 minutes
Cook time: 3 hours 25 minutes
Servings: 10

Ingredients
- 1 cup almond flour
- ⅓ cup coconut flour
- 1 cup black olives, halved
- 1 cup green olives, halved
- 1 tsp. baking powder
- 1 tsp. active dry yeast
- ⅓ cup unsweetened almond milk
- ⅔ cup shredded mozzarella cheese
- ¼ cup melted unsalted butter
- ¼ cup chopped green onions
- ⅓ cup mayonnaise

Directions
1. In a bowl, combine the almond flour, coconut flour, mozzarella cheese, green onions, olives, and baking powder.
2. In another bowl, combine the milk, mayonnaise, and butter.
3. Add everything in the bread machine, including the yeast, according to bread machine recommendation.
4. Select the Basic bread and press Start.
5. Remove the bread once done.
6. Cool, slice, and serve.

Nutritional Facts Per Serving
- Calories: 134
- Fat: 6.8g
- Carb: 4.2g
- Protein: 12.1g

Goat Cheese Bread

Prep time: 10 minutes
Cook time: 3 hours and 25 minutes
Servings: 10

Ingredients
- 1 ½ cups almond flour
- ¼ tsp. salt
- 2 tsp. fresh thyme, crushed
- ½ cup coconut milk, melted
- 1 tsp. cayenne pepper
- 2 eggs
- 1 tsp. mustard of Dijon
- 1 cup crumbled goat cheese
- 1 tsp. baking powder
- ⅓ cup olive oil
- 1 tsp. active dry yeast

Directions
1. In a bowl, add almond flour, thyme, cayenne pepper, salt, goat cheese, and baking powder.
2. In another bowl, add oil, eggs, milk, and mustard.
3. Add everything in the bread machine, including the yeast, according to bread machine recommendation.
4. Select Basic bread and press Start.
5. Remove the bread when done.
6. Cool, slice, and serve.

Nutritional Facts Per Serving
- Calories: 134
- Fat: 6.8g
- Carb: 4.2g
- Protein: 12.1g

Pumpkin Pecan Bread

Prep time: 10 minutes
Cook time: 3 hours 25 minutes
Servings: 16

Ingredients
- ½ cup almond milk
- ½ cup canned pumpkin
- 1 egg
- 2 tbsp. margarine or butter, cut into pieces
- 3 cups bread flour
- 3 tbsp. erythritol, grounded
- 3/4 tsp salt
- ¼ tsp ground nutmeg
- ¼ tsp ground ginger
- 1/8 tsp ground cloves
- 1 tsp active dry yeast or bread machine yeast
- 3/4 cup coarsely chopped pecans

Directions
1. Add everything to the bread machine.
2. Select Basic cycle and press Start.
3. Remove the bread when done.
4. Cool, slice, and serve.

Nutritional Facts Per Serving
- Calories: 159
- Fat: 6g
- Carb: 8g
- Protein: 4g

Ricotta Chive Bread

Prep time: 10 minutes
Cook time: 3 hours 25 minutes
Servings: 10

Ingredients
- 1 cup lukewarm water
- ⅓ cup ricotta cheese
- 1 ½ tsp salt
- 1 tbsp. granulated sugar
- 3 cups almond flour
- ½ cup chopped chives
- 2 ½ tsp instant yeast

Directions
1. Add everything in the bread machine.
2. Select Basic bread and press Start.
3. Remove the bread when done.
4. Cool, slice, and serve.

Nutritional Facts Per Serving
- Calories: 92
- Fat: 8g
- Carb: 7g
- Protein: 3g

Cheese Cauliflower Broccoli Bread

Prep time: 10 minutes
Cook time: 3 hours and 25 minutes
Servings: 12

Ingredients
- ¼ cup water
- 4 tbsp. oil
- 1 egg white
- 1 tsp lemon juice
- ⅔ cup grated cheddar cheese
- 3 tbsp. green onion
- ½ cup broccoli, chopped
- ½ cup cauliflower, chopped
- ½ tsp lemon-pepper seasoning
- 2 cup almond flour
- 1 tsp regular or quick-rising yeast

Directions
1. Add everything to the bread machine pan.
2. Select Basic and press Start.
3. Remove the bread when done.
4. Cool, slice, and serve.

Nutritional Facts Per Serving
- Calories: 156
- Fat: 7.4g
- Carb: 7g
- Protein: 4.9g

Anise Almond Bread

Prep time: 10 minutes
Cook time: 3 hours and 25 minutes
Servings: 12

Ingredients
- 3/4 cup water
- ¼ cup egg substitute
- ¼ cup butter or margarine, softened
- ¼ cup granulated sugar
- ½ tsp salt
- 3 cup almond butter
- 1 tsp anise seed
- 2 tsp active dry yeast
- ½ cup almonds, chopped small

Directions
1. Add everything to the machine pan except almonds.
2. Select Basic bread and press Start.
3. Add the almonds after the beep.
4. Remove the bread when done.
5. Cool, slice, and serve.

Nutritional Facts Per Serving
- Calories: 78
- Fat: 4g
- Carb: 7g
- Protein: 3g

Cinnamon Cake

Prep time: 10 minutes
Cook time: 3 hours and 30 minutes
Servings: 12

Ingredients
- ½ cup erythritol
- ½ cup butter
- ½ tbsp. vanilla extract
- 1 ¾ cups almond flour
- 1 ½ tsp baking powder
- 1 ½ tsp cinnamon
- ¼ tsp sea salt
- 1 ½ cup carrots, grated
- 1 cup pecans, chopped

Directions
1. Grate carrots and place in a food processor.
2. Add in the rest of the ingredients, except the pecans, and process until well-incorporated.
3. Fold in pecans.
4. Pour mixture into bread machine pan.
5. Set bread machine to bake.
6. When baking is complete, remove from bread machine and transfer to a cooling rack.

Allow to cool completely before slicing. (You can also top with a sugar-free cream cheese frosting, see "Red Velvet Cake" recipe).

You can store it for up to 5 days in the refrigerator.

Nutritional Facts Per Serving
- Calories: 350
- Fat: 34g
- Carb: 8g
- Protein: 7g

Collagen Keto Bread

Prep time: 5 minutes
Cook time: 3 hours and 25 minutes
Servings: 12

Ingredients
- ½ cup collagen protein, unflavored grass-fed
- 6 tbsp. almond flour
- 5 eggs
- 1 tbsp. coconut oil, melted
- 1 tsp baking powder
- 1 tsp xanthan gum
- ¼ tsp Himalayan pink salt

Directions
1. Pour all wet ingredients into bread machine bread pan.
2. Add dry ingredients to the bread machine pan.
3. Set bread machine to the gluten-free setting
4. When the bread is done, remove bread machine pan from the bread machine.
5. Let cool slightly before transferring to a cooling rack.

The bread can be stored for up to 4 days on the counter and for up to 3 months in the freezer.

Nutritional Facts Per Serving
- Calories: 77
- Fat: 14g
- Carb: 6g
- Protein: 5g

APPENDIX : RECIPES INDEX

3-Seed Bread 16

A

Almond Butter Bread 40
Almond Meal Bread 14
American Cheese Beer Bread 75
Anise Almond Bread 100
Avocado Bread 71

B

Bacon and Cheddar Bread 21
Bacon Bread 84
Banana Bread 33
Banana Bread 70
Basil Cheese Bread 77
Blueberry Bread 45
Blueberry Bread 68
Buttermilk Bread 56

C

Cauliflower and Garlic Bread 13
Cauliflower Bread 85
Cheddar and Herb Bread 27
Cheese and Bacon Bread 29
Cheese Cauliflower Broccoli Bread 99
Cheese Sausage Bread 78
Cheesy Garlic Bread 17
Chocolate and Pistachio Bread 54
Chocolate Bread 46
Chocolate Bread 51
Chocolate Bread 69
Chocolate Zucchini Bread 41
Chocolate, Mixed Berry, and Nuts Bread 59
Chocolate, Mixed Berry, and Nuts Cake 36
Cinnamon Bread 37
Cinnamon Cake 101
Coconut Milk Bread 35
Collagen Keto Bread 102
Cottage Cheese Bread 92
Cranberry and Orange Bread 44
Cream Cheese Bread 87
Cream Cheese Bread 11
Cumin Bread 18

D

Date and Walnut Bread 76
Delicious Cranberry and Cream Cheese 50
Delicious Lemon Bread 47
Delicious Pumpkin Bread 49
Dill and Cheddar Bread 24

F

Feta Oregano Bread 91
French Ham Bread 79

G

Garlic and Dill Bread 58
Garlic Bread 88
Gingerbread Cake 72
Goat Cheese Bread 96

H

Herb Bread 86
Holiday Bread 74

I

Italian Mozzarella and Cream Cheese Bread 25

J

Jalapeño Cheese Bread 23

K

Keto Almond Pumpkin Quick Bread 31
Keto Apple Bread 52
Keto Basil Parmesan Slices 32
Keto Basil Parmesan Slices 82
Keto Onion Bread 80

L

Lemon and Blueberry Bread 61
Lemon Bread 73
Lemon Poppy Seed Bread 12
Lemon Raspberry Loaf 38
Low-Carb Cranberry and Walnut Bread 53
Low-Carb Date and Walnut Bread 55
Low-Carb Pound Cake Loaf 63
Low-Carb Wheat-Style Bread 60

M

Macadamia Nut Bread 15

O

Olive Bread 22
Olive Cheese Bread 95
Orange Bread 62

P

Parmesan Cheddar Bread 93
Peach Cake Bread 57
Pepper Cheddar Bread 94
Pumpkin Bread 30
Pumpkin Bread 42
Pumpkin Pecan Bread 97

R

Raspberry Bread 67
Red Velvet Cake 64
Ricotta Chive Bread 98
Rosemary Bread 19

S

Scandinavian Bread 90
Sesame and Flax Seed Bread 20
Sesame Bread 89

Sourdough Dough 26
Strawberry Bread 43
Strawberry Bread 48
Sweet Avocado Bread 34

T

Tomato Bread 81

V

Vegan Keto Bread 65
Vegetable Loaf 28

W

Walnut Bread 39

Z

Zucchini Bread 66
Zucchini Bread 83

CPSIA information can be obtained
at www.ICGtesting.com
Printed in the USA
BVHW052047060421
604208BV00005BA/911